AF414309

GUIDE TO THE GUIDELINES

Volume 1

Bread and Butter GI

*A vignette-based journey through the ACG
clinical practice guidelines*

Brennan Spiegel, MD, MSHS, FACG
and
Hetal A. Karsan, MD, FACG

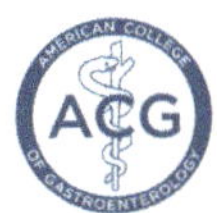

Address editorial correspondence to:
American College of Gastroenterology
11333 Woodglen Drive, Suite 100
North Bethesda, MD 20852, USA

Contact the American College of Gastroenterology
Phone: 301-263-9028
Email: info@gi.org
Online store: https://members.gi.org/store/

All rights are reserved, including those for text and data mining, AI training, and similar technologies. No part of this book may be used or reproduced, stored in a retrieval system, or transmitted in any form or by any means, electronic, mechanical, photocopying, recording or otherwise, without the written permission of the American College of Gastroenterology or the authors.

© 2023 American College of Gastroenterology

ISBN: 979-8-218-37004-6

Contents

KNOW YOUR GUIDELINES!

"What do the ACG guidelines say?"

If you're a practicing gastroenterologist or hepatologist, then that's an excellent question. It's a question you probably ask yourself every day you are in clinic. It's a question that determines how best to diagnose, treat, and deliver the highest quality care for patients with digestive diseases. Bottom line is this: you really must know the guidelines!

Of course, the best way to know the guidelines is to read them. As of this writing, the American College of Gastroenterology (ACG) has published over 70 guidelines covering diseases of the esophagus, to disorders the anorectum, to, well, just about everywhere else between the poles of the alimentary canal. These documents are pure gold. They lay out, in evidence-based splendor, the key recommendations that govern clinical practice in our field. They are required reading.

But let's be fair about something. Reading through 70+ guidelines encompassing well over 4,000 pages of text and drawing from over 10,000 citations is not easy sledding. By the time you reach the end of the guidelines you probably need to start over because (a) you forgot some things, (b) the guidelines are periodically revised, and (c) new guidelines are constantly in the works.

That's why we wrote this book. As a former Editor-in-Chief of *The American Journal of Gastroenterology* (B.S.) and former Editor of the Journal's "Red Section" (H.K.), we have observed a strong desire among clinicians to learn the guidelines in efficient, accessible, and fun ways. We discovered that our most popular Journal podcasts were those about the ACG guidelines and the most successful Red Section columns were authored by senior clinicians who interpreted the guidelines through an expert lens shaped by years of practice.

We got to thinking: wouldn't it be handy to have a "guide to the guidelines" that digested (pun intended) the thousand pages of ACG documents into a concise, entertaining, and useful review of the most salient pearls and insights? We imagined a resource that would reflect the accessible style of our AJG podcasts with the pragmatic lessons in the most popular Red Section columns. Also, because clinicians learn by example, we figured that a vignette-based journey through the guidelines would bring the ACG material to life in ways that a typical textbook might fall short (peeps love to learn from vignettes). That led to the book you are reading now.

Here's how we structured *Guide to the Guidelines*, which we'll call *G2G* for short: We mapped each of the ACG guidelines into one of 3 major topics. Each topic composes one of 3 volumes for the G2G series. You are now reading Volume I, titled *Bread and Butter GI*. In this volume, we cover common luminal topics that comprise everyday practice for the general gastroenterologist. In Chapter 1, *Gut Feelings*, we summarize all the neurogastroenterology and motility guidelines, including irritable bowel syndrome (IBS), small intestinal bacterial overgrowth (SIBO), dyspepsia, constipation, gastroparesis, and benign anorectal disorders. Chapter 2, *Down the Hatch*, reviews the key esophagus guidelines including gastro-esophageal reflux disease (GERD), Barrett's esophagus, esophageal eosinophilia, and achalasia. Finally, in Chapter 3, *Lumps and Bumps,* we cover prevention and treatment of luminal tumors, including colorectal cancer screening and surveillance guidelines, GI polyposis syndromes, hereditary GI cancer syndromes, gastric premalignant conditions, and submucosal masses. All mnemonics used were designed by B. Spiegel.

The forthcoming Volume II of the G2G series, titled *GI Infection, Inflammation, and Bleeding* will cover the inflammatory bowel diseases including Crohn disease (yes, it's called "Crohn disease," not "Crohn's disease"), ulcerative colitis, and celiac disease. It will also review the GI infection guidelines, including *Clostridioides difficile, Helicobacter pylori*, and acute diarrheal infections. Volume II will conclude by summarizing the guidelines on upper GI and ulcer bleeding, small bowel bleeding, lower GI bleeding, management of anticoagulants and antiplatelet drugs during acute GI bleeding, and colon ischemia. It's gonna be a banger!

In Volume III, we will leave the main luminal highway and head towards the extraluminal onramps, including the pancreas and biliary system. There, we will review the ACG guidelines on biliary strictures, use of ERCP and EUS, pancreatic cysts, pancreatitis, and primary sclerosing cholangitis. Finally, we end with that big organ up top: the liver. We'll review the guidelines on alcoholic liver diseases, focal liver lesions, hemochromatosis, acute liver failure, hepatic and mesenteric circulation, abnormal liver tests, drug induced liver injury, pregnancy and liver disease, and nutrition in liver disease. Yep, that's a lot of guidelines!

Each G2G chapter includes carefully selected vignettes designed to illustrate key concepts from the guidelines, followed by a conversation-style discussion written to keep you awake and alert. As you read these discussions, you'll notice that we highlight specific points along the margin that we think are especially noteworthy. Then, following each chapter, we provide multiple-choice questions to test your knowledge of the material. We prepared questions that highlight information we believe is most vital to ensure high quality care, as judged by our nearly fifty years of combined experience managing GI and liver patients in both academic and private practice settings (yikes, we're getting old). We also worked with the authors of each ACG guideline to ensure our treatment of their document is accurate. We hope you find the discussions and questions to be both enjoyable and useful.

We also might throw in some jokes from time-to-time. You might not think they are as funny as we do; we'll see. We also might use words like "pee" and "poo" because we also think that's funny. You'll have to roll with it.

A quick word on what this book is not. First and foremost, *it is not a substitute for reading the guidelines.* The best way to learn the guidelines is to read the guidelines. We could not cover every fact in every guideline or else we'd just have bound them into one fat tome. That's not the point of this resource. Instead, our goal is to augment the original documents with an engaging and interactive precis, not to unload a comprehensive restatement of the original works. This book is also not designed to be a mere Cliff's Notes version of the guidelines. If that were the case, then we'd just re-write the original text using one-tenth the number of words (or worse, just ask ChatGPT to summarize the guidelines, which it can do in mere seconds). Nah, this ain't no AI-written book. Instead, this is a vignette-driven exploration of the guidelines dosed with ample interpretation from years of clinical experience, pragmatic tips on how to apply the guidelines to your practice, and answers to common questions raised but not directly addressed by the guidelines. G2G is also not specifically designed for board review. There are many other resources to prepare for the gastroenterology board examination, including an entire book series we've previously written (feel free to check those out separately) and many others. Finally, this book is not a substitute for other ACG resources, such as educational videos on ACG Universe, CME questions from the ACG Annual Postgraduate Course, or multiple-choice questions that accompany guidelines in *The American Journal of Gastroenterology.* Instead, we prepared a standalone resource designed to augment other offerings in a way that is novel and (we hope...) valuable to practicing members of ACG, trainees, and other clinicians seeking to reinforce their knowledge of the ACG guidelines.

One last note: Because the ACG guidelines are constantly revised and updated, the book you are now reading will eventually become outdated. In fact, it might *already* be outdated! That's the nature of guidelines. It's important to keep up with the latest recommendations because they often change meaningfully as scientific evidence emerges. We will continue to update this book to ensure it remains modern and accurate.

We hope you enjoy reading G2G as much as we enjoyed writing it. If nothing else, preparing this resource in partnership with the ACG helped us learn the guidelines and we trust it will help you, too.

Brennan Spiegel, MD, MSHS, FACG
Professor of Medicine and Public Health
Gourrich Chair in Digital Health Ethics
Director of Health Services Research,
Cedars-Sinai
Director, Cedars-Sinai Master's Degree
Program in Health Delivery Science

Hetal A. Karsan, MD, FACG
Chair of Credentials Committee, ACG
International Governor, ACG
Chair of Medical Education,
United Digestive
Adjunct Professor of Medicine, Emory
University

Chapter One

Gut Feelings

Neurogastroentrology & Motility Guidelines

Do you know the difference between small intestinal bacterial overgrowth (SIBO) and intestinal methanogen overgrowth (IMO)? How do gut archaea differ from gut bacteria? Not sure? Well, you're not alone. Unless you keep up with the latest gut microbiome guidelines, some of this might sound unfamiliar. How about this: do you feel comfortable interpreting hydrogen breath tests? And when should you use lactulose vs glucose for breath testing? Does it matter? You may be scratching your head. Or maybe not (in which case, feel free to skip ahead, smarty pants!).

In this chapter, we'll cover the ACG neurogastroenterology and motility guidelines. This not only includes the guidelines on SIBO, but also the guidelines on irritable bowel syndrome (IBS), dyspepsia, constipation, gastroparesis, and benign anorectal disorders. These topics comprise the "bread and butter" of general gastroenterology practice. You've just got to know these ACG guidelines. Let's get started with that SIBO vs IMO thing.

Case 1.1: Breath Testing for IBS

A 28-year-old woman presents with a 10-year history of constipation marked by passage of infrequent and hard stools, a sense of incomplete evacuation, painful defecation, and associated bloating and lower abdominal pain that occur daily. The pain improves with passing a bowel movement. She does not report weight loss, rectal bleeding, or other alarm symptoms. She is not anemic and other lab tests have been unrevealing. She was diagnosed as having IBS with constipation (IBS-C) and received various treatments over several years, including fiber, laxatives, guanylate cyclase C agonists, neuromodulators, and gut-directed psychotherapy. However, her constipation and bloating have persisted with only partial benefit from treatment. A lactulose breath test is now obtained with the results show in **Figure 1.1**.

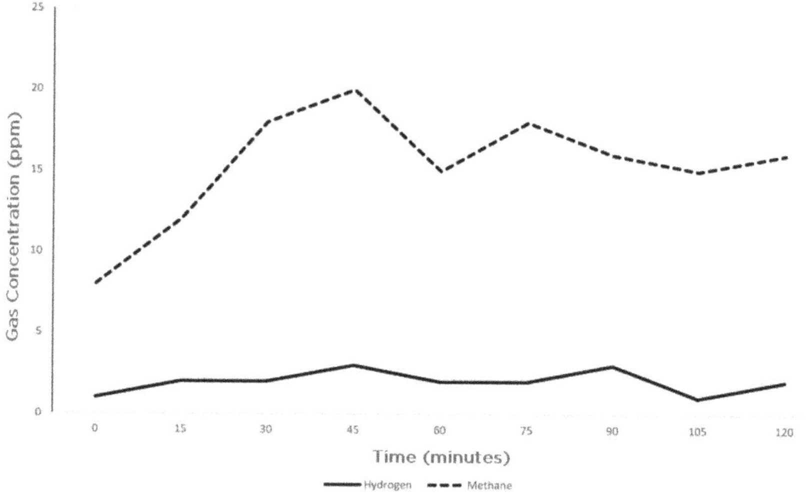

Figure 1.1. Results of lactulose breath test.

Know your guidelines!

1. How do you interpret this breath test?
2. How should you treat this gas pattern?

Case 1.1: What do the guidelines say?

Source: ACG 2020 SIBO Guidelines

Bloating. Diarrhea. Constipation. Distension. Bloating. Diarrhea. Constipation. Distension. Bloating...

Yep, welcome to the world of outpatient gastroenterology. If you've spent even an hour in a GI clinic, then you know these are among the most common symptoms known to humankind. That's why the ACG SIBO guidelines are so useful; they help us better understand these common and bothersome symptoms and offer a rigorous framework for diagnosis and treatment.

Let's break down the case. This patient meets the Rome IV criteria for IBS, meaning she has recurrent abdominal pain ≥1 day per week for at least the previous 3 months that is associated with 2 or more of the following: (1) related to defecation; (2) associated with a change in stool frequency; (3) associated with a change in stool form or appearance.[1] The lack of alarm features is consistent with IBS and the presence of constipation—marked by infrequent and hard stools with incomplete evacuation—means IBS-C is a good diagnosis. As an aside, earlier versions of the Rome criteria allowed patients to have either abdominal pain *or discomfort*, but the term "discomfort" proved to be non-specific, so now we just go with "pain"—not discomfort.

The issue here is this patient already received several evidence-based treatments including pharmacotherapies and gut-directed behavioral therapies. We'll talk about IBS treatments later, but the point here is that her symptoms continued despite treatment. In this instance, it is reasonable to perform a breath test to screen for SIBO since bacterial overgrowth occurs in around 35% of IBS patients and antibiotics are often effective at reducing symptom burden.[2] More on antibiotics soon.

Let's take a moment to define SIBO. Simply put, SIBO occurs when the small intestine is colonized by an excessive amount of predominantly gram negative aerobic and anerobic bacteria that are normally found in the large intestine.[3] Because these gram-negative buggers ferment carbohydrates and produce gas, patients with SIBO may experience GI symptoms, including bloating, distention, diarrhea, and constipation. Whereas the old definition of SIBO was $\geq 10^5$ colony-forming units per milliliter (CFU/mL) in a duodenal or jejunal aspirate, both the ACG guidelines and the North American Consensus on breath testing[4] determined that the $\geq 10^5$ threshold is too high and now suggest a lower threshold of $\geq 10^3$ CFU/mL. That said, it's worth noting that very few people diagnose SIBO using a small bowel aspirate since it is expensive, technically cumbersome, and invasive. Instead, the ACG guidelines recommend performing a breath test as a less invasive, cheaper, and better tolerated surrogate for SIBO, even if it's not a true gold standard like culturing small bowel aspirate.

Before we get into the details of performing and interpreting a breath test, here's a question to ponder: Should all IBS patients receive a breath test? The ACG offers this purposefully noncommittal guidance: "We suggest the use of breath testing for the diagnosis of SIBO in patients with IBS." So, not a clear-cut "yes," but a suggested yes. We describe the guideline statement as "noncommittal" because it is accompanied by a "conditional" recommendation, meaning the level of evidence is very low. What this means, in practice, is that you are under no obligation to routinely order a breath test in allcomers with IBS, and, truth be told, virtually nobody does that in practice. In fact, the utility of routine breath testing has been questioned.[5]

However, there are special situations that boost the chances of SIBO and lower the threshold for ordering a breath test. This patient, for example, has not responded to evidence-based IBS therapies, thus raising the possibility of untreated SIBO. Although not

Know the causes of SIBO…there's a bunch of them

mentioned in this case, other situations that should trigger your SIBO Spidey-sense include diabetes, hypochlorhydria (e.g. high-dose PPIs, atrophic gastritis), connective tissue disorders (e.g., scleroderma, Ehlers Danlos Syndrome [EDS]), malabsorption conditions (e.g. pancreatic insufficiency, celiac disease), mechanical causes (e.g. small bowel tumors, volvulus), opioids, small bowel diverticulosis, Crohn disease, an incompetent ileocecal valve, history of luminal surgery (especially blind loops), chronic liver disease, immunodeficiencies (e.g. HIV, common variable immunodeficiency, selective IgA deficiency, etc.), thyroid disease, and amyloidosis. Is that a hard list to memorize? Well, here's a fun fact: we realized that all those SIBO culprits conveniently spell out the word "DYSMOTILITY," which is the underlying mechanism for many cases of SIBO. Check it out!

Diabetes
h**Y**pochlorhydria
Scleroderma
Malabsorption / **M**echanical causes
Opioids
Tics / **T**issue Issues (e.g., EDS)
IBS / **I**BD / **I**ncompetent IC valve
Luminal surgery / **L**iver disease
Immunodeficiency
Thyroid disease
am**Y**loidosis

Figure 1.2: A memory aid to learn the causes of SIBO. They conveniently spell out the word "DYSMOTILITY" (more or less).

Okay, so let's say you suspect SIBO and now want to order a breath test. Does it matter whether it's a lactulose or glucose-based breath test? What's the difference, anyway? For starters, know that the ACG guidelines do not make a recommendation about which substrate to use; *both are acceptable*, so long as you use 75g of glucose or 10g of lactulose, each with 1 cup of water (~250mL). That said, there are important differences between using glucose vs lactulose. Glucose is rapidly absorbed in the proximal small bowel, meaning that it does not normally pass into the colon. In contrast, lactulose is not absorbed, meaning that all of it passes into the colon. If there is an early rise in breath hydrogen or methane after ingesting glucose, then it means the substrate was fermented in the small bowel—not in the colon—which is consistent with SIBO. In contrast, an early rise in breath hydrogen or methane after ingesting lactulose might indicate the substrate encountered overgrowth in the small bowel, but it could also mean the lactulose quickly reached the colon where bacterial fermentation yielded a false positive result. For that reason, some argue the lactulose breath test is really a measure of oro-cecal transit time rather than a true measure of SIBO,[6] whereas the glucose breath test might be more specific for SIBO because glucose doesn't readily pass into the large bowel. That said, the ACG guidelines indicate that both tests are similar in terms of sensitivity and specificity, so picking between substrates is mainly based on local preference and expertise.

Now, to answer the questions in this vignette we need to understand how to interpret breath tests. Good news: the rules are the same for glucose and lalctulose; in both cases the ACG guidelines indicate that a rise in breath hydrogen of $\geq$20 parts per million (ppm) from baseline within 90 minutes <u>or</u> a rise in breath methane of $\geq$10 ppm at any time during the test is considered "positive." You might ask, *positive for what?* And that's where things get a little more interesting. An early rise in breath hydrogen after ingesting glucose

ACG is cool with either glucose or lactulose for breath testing; it's your call

For GHBT use 75 g glucose; for LHBT use 10 g lactulose

Glucose is absorbed in proximal small bowel. Lactulose is not absorbed

Positive breath test:

• $\geq$ 20 ppm rise in hydrogen within 90 min, or…

• $\geq$ 10 ppm rise in methane at any time

or lactulose suggests SIBO. But when breath methane rises it suggests "IMO," meaning "intestinal methanogen overgrowth."

So, what's the difference between SIBO and IMO? The answer comes down to understanding the difference between hydrogen-producing bacteria, sulfate-reducing bacteria, and methanogenic archaea. It's not that complicated, but if you've never thought about this before, then it might take a second to understand what's happening deep down in that nutty microbiome.

Here's the deal: When a carbohydrate like lactulose or glucose encounters gram negative bacteria in the small intestine, it generates hydrogen gas, or H_2. So far, so good. From there, single-celled archaea, *which are not technically bacteria*, use the hydrogen to form methane, or CH_4. Thus, when there is $\geq$ 10 ppm of breath methane measured after ingesting glucose or lactulose, it means there is overgrowth of methanogenic archaea, which the ACG guidelines call IMO. The most common type of IMO-producing archaea is *Methanobrevibacter smithii*. Since archaea like *M. smithii* are not bacteria, it doesn't make sense to use the term SIBO since the "B" in SIBO stands for "bacteria," whereas the problem with IMO is overgrowth of methanogenic archaea. In contrast, if there is a lot of hydrogen gas or hydrogen-sulfide (H_2S) gas in the breath, then it indicates SIBO. **Figure 1.3** is from the ACG SIBO guidelines and demonstrates how the gas from hydrogen-producing bacteria can be transformed into either methane, on the one hand, or hydrogen-sulfide, on the other. It all depends on whether there is an overgrowth of methanogenic archaea or sulfate-reducing bacteria. Pretty interesting.

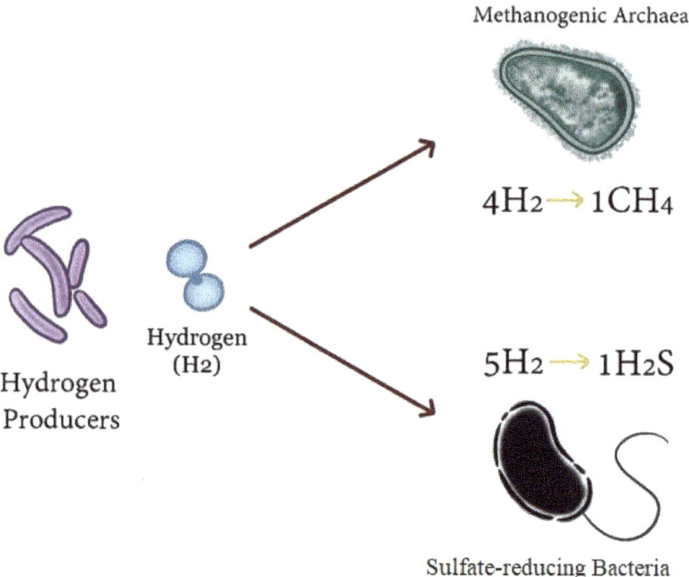

Figure 1.3: Bacterial overgrowth in the small intestine produces hydrogen gas in the setting of a carbohydrate load. The hydrogen gas, in turn, feeds archaea that can form methane gas or, conversely, feed sulfate-reducing bacteria that generate hydrogen sulfide gas. Image from ACG SIBO guidelines.[3]

Methane slows intestinal transit, leading to constipation

This is not just an academic distinction. The difference between SIBO and IMO has clinical implications shown in **Table 1.1**. When there is overgrowth of methanogenic archaea, the resulting methane slows intestinal transit and can lead to constipation. In this vignette, the breath test reveals evidence of IMO, but not SIBO, because there is a rise in breath methane but not breath hydrogen. In contrast, if the breath hydrogen had risen $\geq$ 20 ppm within 90 minutes, then it would have indicated SIBO. When hydrogen gas is present, it can be further characterized as pure hydrogen vs hydrogen-sulfide, where H_2S tends to correlate more with diarrhea than constipation.

Production of H_2S gas is associated with diarrhea

Table 1.1: *Small intestinal bacterial overgrowth vs intestinal methanogen overgrowth.*

Type of Overgrowth	Gas Produced	Symptom	Antibiotics Recommended by ACG Guidelines
SIBO	Hydrogen	Not correlated with a specific symptom	Amoxicillin-clavulanate (875mg BID) Ciprofloxacin (500mg BID) Doxycycline (100mg QD to BID) Metronidazole (250mg TID) Neomycin (500mg BID) Norfloxacin (400mg QD) Rifaximin (550mg TID) Tetracycline (250mg QID) Trimethoprim-sulfamethoxazole (160mg/800mg BID)
	Hydrogen Sulfide	Diarrhea	
IMO	Methane	Constipation	Consider combination therapy with rifaximin and neomycin

Whereas SIBO can be treated by a wide range of antibiotics, IMO may not respond as well to a single antibiotic. Although not a formal recommendation, the ACG guidelines refer to literature showing that combination therapy with rifaximin and neomycin may be most effective in treating IBS-C in patients with IMO.[7] Bear in mind that neomycin can, on rare occasions, be toxic to the kidneys and inner ear, so always use your clinical judgment when prescribing this agent.

Consider treating IMO with a combination of rifaximin and neomycin (or whatever insurance will cover!)

By the way, do you need to check a breath test before starting an antibiotic for IBS? No. The IBS guidelines are silent on whether breath testing should be performed before treating with antibiotics[8] and the original rifaximin trials did not require breath testing prior to initiating therapy. However, the guidelines point out that rifaximin is more effective in people with a positive vs negative breath test (56% vs 25% response, respectively).[9]

Rifaximin is more effective in patients with a positive HBT

Antibiotics aren't the only way to treat SIBO or IMO. The ACG guidelines also discuss the role of diet manipulation as another strategy to modify intestinal pathogens. A diet low in fermentable products, such as fiber, alcohol sugars, inulin, and sweeteners like sucralose, are useful to consider although data supporting diet manipulation remain limited. The low FODMAP diet, discussed later in this chapter, is mainly validated for use in IBS rather than SIBO or IMO, and currently the quality of evidence for the low FODMAP diet, even when used for IBS, is "very low" according to ACG guidelines. Nonetheless, for IBS patients concerned about using antibiotics, it is reasonable to recommend a diet low in fermentable products as a non-pharmacological alternative.

What about probiotics? We'll make this part short. The guidelines just don't currently recommend probiotics either for IBS in general, or for IBS related to SIBO. In fact, one controlled study indicated that probiotics have potential to *cause* SIBO,[10] suggesting that use of probiotics is not straightforward and may even cause harm. The same applies to fecal microbiota transplant, or FMT. Currently, there is no role for using FMT in IBS, SIBO, or IMO, and the ACG "strongly" recommends against its use for all these conditions.

Bottom line with this case: the breath test reveals IMO. It would be reasonable to treat with rifaximin and neomycin if there are no contraindications.

Case 1.2: Diagnostic testing for IBS

A 32-year-old woman has experienced a decade of recurrent abdominal pain, diarrhea, and bloating. She was diagnosed with IBS-D while in college but has never received treatment. She has no stool incontinence, rectal bleeding, weight loss, nausea, vomiting, fevers, sweats, or other alarm features. There is no other significant past medical history. She has no allergies, takes no medications, and denies use of illicit substances. Examination reveals no alarm features and is positive only for mild left lower quadrant tenderness. Her primary care provider obtained a complete blood count that did not reveal anemia or other abnormalities. Electrolyte and liver tests were normal, but no other recent laboratory, imaging, or endoscopic tests have been performed.

Know your guidelines!

The table below provides a list of diagnostic tests that are sometimes ordered to rule out IBS mimics. For each one, check off whether the ACG IBS guidelines recommend, or don't recommend, checking that test routinely for a patient like the one described in this vignette.

Table 1.2. *Yay or Nay? For each of these diagnostic tests, select whether it is recommended or not by the ACG IBS clinical guidelines.*
Go ahead and fill it out, at least in your head, before reading on.

Diagnostic Test	Recommended	Not Recommended
Serologic testing for celiac disease		
Fecal calprotectin		
C-reactive protein		
Erythrocyte sedimentation rate		
Colonoscopy with biopsy		
Fecal ova & parasites		
Stool testing for enteric pathogens		
Food allergy testing		

Case 1.2: What do the guidelines say?

Source: ACG 2021 IBS Guidelines

Before diving into the ACG IBS guidelines, let's start with some practical questions: Do you believe that IBS is a diagnosis of exclusion? If so, what tests must be negative before you are willing to confidently diagnose IBS? In contrast, do you feel comfortable diagnosing IBS even with minimal diagnostic testing, so long as your patient meets Rome criteria[1] and, say, doesn't have anemia? Just how much testing is enough? The IBS guidelines have something to say about all these questions, but it's worth a moment to think about your own beliefs and practice patterns.

Way back in 2010, one of us led a study to examine whether clinicians really believe that IBS is a diagnosis of exclusion.[11] The ACG guidelines stated then—*as they do now*—that IBS should *not* be considered a diagnosis of exclusion and that clinicians should instead make a positive diagnosis using the Rome criteria with minimal testing. Yet, many clinicians remain concerned about missing serious conditions lurking beneath the veneer of an IBS diagnosis. We checked to see how docs approached diagnostic testing in IBS. And what did we find? Well... let's just say most were non-plussed by the guidelines. They tested. A lot.

Whereas "IBS experts" in the study were less likely to consider IBS a diagnosis of exclusion and ordered 50% fewer tests than community practitioners, most providers believed IBS should only be diagnosed after exclusionary testing; they rated most of the tests in Table 1.2 as "appropriate." In other words, there was a big disconnect between IBS experts and community providers. Why the difference? Medicolegal concerns? Lack of familiarity with the guidelines? Lack of agreement with the guidelines? We weren't exactly sure.

Fast forward to 2021 when the latest ACG IBS guidelines were published.[8] In the decade between our study and release of the latest guidelines, there has been more (and more...) evidence building that excessive testing is low yield and expensive. Although there are cases where extra testing is warranted (and we will cover that in a bit), most of the time it's best to minimize testing, make a positive diagnosis, and jump straight to treatment.

With that background, let's see what the ACG guidelines say about each of the tests listed in Table 1.2. We'll go through them briefly, starting with tests the guidelines recommend, and then covering tests that aren't recommended.

Tests Recommended for IBS

Serologic testing for celiac disease: Of all the tests you might order to evaluate a patient with IBS, testing for celiac disease is among the most important and strongly recommended by the ACG. The reasons are obvious. Untreated celiac disease can have serious consequences, including neuropsychiatric symptoms, autoimmune comorbidities, infertility, and of course, GI malignancies and lymphoma. So, we can't let IBS patients go years receiving unnecessary and ineffective treatments only to learn they had celiac disease all along. That would be bad. Meta-analysis reveals that 2.6% of IBS patients are seropositive for celiac disease, which is higher than the 1.4% background prevalence of celiac seropositivity in North America.[12] When pooling studies from across the world, IBS patients are 4.5 times more likely to have underlying biopsy-proven celiac disease compared to population controls.[13] As expected, celiac seropositivity is higher for those with IBS-D (5.7%) compared to IBS-M (3.4%) and IBS-C (2.1%).[13] Notice that even IBS-C patients can have celiac disease. The ACG guidelines recommend screening IBS patients with immunoglobulin A (IgA) tissue transglutaminase (TTG) and quantitative IgA level (since selective IgA deficiency occurs in 2% of celiac patients which, if present, causes a false negative anti-TTG IgA). We also showed years ago that testing for celiac disease in IBS is cost-effective.[14] Positive tests should be followed by upper endoscopy with at least 6 biopsies from the duodenum, including the duodenal bulb. More on the ACG celiac disease guidelines coming in Volume II of the G2G series.

Inflammatory markers: Just like we don't want to overlook celiac disease, we also don't want to miss other inflammatory bowel diseases (IBD) misdiagnosed as IBS, such as Crohn disease or ulcerative colitis. The prevalence of IBD among people diagnosed with IBS is low at around 1% or less.[15] But... (and this is a big "but"), for IBS patients with 5 or more years of symptoms the risk of IBD rises up to 5x higher than controls.[16,17] We call this the IBS/IBD *rule of 5s.* Keep that rule in mind when an IBS patient continues with symptoms despite receiving evidence-based treatments. Because there is some overlap between IBS and IBD, the ACG guidelines *strongly* recommend checking either a fecal calprotectin (fCal) or fecal lactoferrin (FL) along with a C-reactive protein (CRP). Both fecal tests are around 90% accurate at discriminating IBS from IBD.[18,19] Of note, measuring erythrocyte sedimentation rate (ESR) is commonly performed but does not accurately discriminate between IBS and IBD, whereas CRP does a better job.[20]

Tests *Not* Recommended for IBS

Colonoscopy with biopsy: We all agree that colonoscopy is indicated for age-appropriate colorectal cancer screening and we'll cover that in depth later in Chapter 3 of this book. An IBS patient who is 45 years or older is eligible for colonoscopy independent of having IBS. Similarly, a patient with alarm features, such as unintended weight loss, rectal bleeding, or iron deficiency anemia, should also be referred for colonoscopy regardless of IBS status. The question here is whether someone young without alarm features, such as the 32-year-old patient with IBS in the vignette, should undergo diagnostic colonoscopy. The ACG guidelines are clear: *nope.* This is based upon studies revealing a low diagnostic yield of colonoscopy for young, otherwise healthy patients with IBS. It is exceeding rare, for example, to find a colon cancer explaining IBS symptoms (0.1% risk in one study cited by the guidelines, where all cancers occurred in patients >50 years old).[21] What about missing IBD? Isn't that a reason to do a colonoscopy? Well, if you're looking for IBD, then you should rely upon the noninvasive fCal and FL tests we discussed earlier; there is no additional need for colonoscopy. What about this: doesn't a negative colonoscopy put patients at ease and help them feel better? Isn't it like giving them a warranty on their colon? Well... not really. Years ago, one of us looked at this question and found no relationship between a negative colonoscopy and the patient feeling reassured or having improved quality of life.[22] Some patients with high neuroticism *might* benefit from a normal colonoscopy, but even they will likely develop new concerns despite receiving a clean bill of colonic health. However, there is one special circumstance when colonoscopy might have a role; we'll cover that scenario shortly. Stay tuned...

Stool testing for bacterial and parasitic organisms: Unless your IBS patient spends a lot of time drinking fresh river water or camping in the mountains (sounds lovely), the chances of finding a parasite like *Giardia* is very small. That's why the ACG guidelines do not recommend testing stool ova and parasites unless there is a high pre-test probability of infection. Similarly, there's a very low chance of finding active *Campylobacter, Salmonella,* or Norwalk virus as the cause of longstanding IBS symptoms. That's why the guidelines also dissuade testing for bacterial or viral pathogens. Of course, bacterial infections can trigger post-infectious IBS

(PI-IBS) in about 11% of cases, but then the organisms disappear, leaving behind IBS without an active infection.[23] *Giardia* can also cause PI-IBS, albeit much less commonly than bacterial pathogens like *Campylobacter.*[24] While we're talking about enteric pathogens, what risk factors increase the chance of developing PI-IBS? Check out **Table 1.3** for the list:

Table 1.3. *Risk factors for PI-IBS.*[25]

Female
Younger age
Prolonged fever
History of anxiety or depression
Longer duration of index infection
Exposed to antibiotics during index infection

Food allergy testing: Undoubtedly, many of your IBS patients will ask whether food is causing their GI symptoms. We'll discuss diet manipulation for IBS later in this chapter, but for now the question is whether you should formally test for food allergies in IBS. Once again, the ACG guidelines say no. Although nearly half of IBS patient report adverse reactions to specific foods, the reactions are rarely a true IgE-mediated food allergy. Food allergy occurs within minutes of ingestion and symptoms are reproducible upon re-challenge with the same food. It would be highly unusual for a food allergy to present only with abdominal pain or diarrhea without any itching, rhinorrhea, laryngospasm, bronchospasm, nausea, vomiting, urticaria, hypotension, or other classic immunologically mediated signs or symptoms. However, if those features are present and reproducible, then the guidelines say it's reasonable to conduct food allergy testing. Otherwise, allergy testing is a low yield and expensive practice not only because the prevalence of food allergies is low among IBS patients, but also because skin prick tests

26

and serum IgE are not very sensitive in the first place. Much more common in IBS is food "intolerance" or food "sensitivity," which are undesirable responses to a culprit food unrelated to an immune response. For example, many IBS patients report a sensitivity to gluten. In the absence of true celiac disease, these patients typically have a non-immunologically mediated sensitivity. In other cases, patients may have a strong response to fructan, a nondigestible carbohydrate prevalent in the Western diet. Intolerances to gluten, fructan, or other fermentable products are very real and should be taken seriously, but they do not mandate formal allergy testing. Nonetheless, this is an area of active research, so time will tell whether allergy testing might prove useful in the future. For now, the guidelines indicate that it is neither effective nor cost-effective to test IBS patients for food allergies.

Okay, but is extra testing *ever* indicated for IBS?

Yes. For sure. Although the ACG guidelines do not support routine use of most tests (other than celiac serology, fCal, LF, and CRP), sometimes we need to dig deeper. The guidelines don't address this point directly, but we want to offer some pragmatic thoughts about patients with persistent IBS symptoms. For example, what if you have a patient with longstanding IBS symptoms despite many unsuccessful rounds of evidence-based treatments? What if they burn through medication after medication, don't respond to dietary modifications, or fail to respond to gut-directed psychotherapies? Should you just throw in the towel and give up? Heck no! When a patient doesn't follow the script and has years of persistent or severe symptoms despite treatment, then you toss the script and start thinking beyond the guidelines. You've got to think of the wolf in sheep's clothing that might masquerade as IBS. What are those masqueraders? Here's a list to consider: acute intermittent porphyria (AIP); neuroendocrine tumors (e.g. carcinoid,

VIPomas); disaccharidase deficiencies (e.g. lactase or sucrase-isomaltase deficiency); SIBO; microscopic colitis; bile acid diarrhea; Ehlers-Danlos Syndrome, and eosinophilic GI disorders, among others. These "invisible" diagnoses might be hidden under the façade of IBS, unrevealed and untreated. If that list is hard to keep in mind, just remember they spell out "INVISIBLE," which is exactly what these conditions will remain unless and until you look for them. Check out **Figure 1.4**.

A I P

N euroendocrine tumor (*e.g.* carcinoid)

V IPoma

I somaltase / sucrase deficiency

S IBO

m I croscopic colitis

B ile acid diarrhea

L actase deficiency

E osinophilic gastrointestinal diseases

Figure 1.4: A memory aid to learn the rare and potentially unrevealed causes of "IBS" in a patient with longstanding symptoms despite usual therapies. They conveniently spell out the word "INVISIBLE" (okay, we broke out VIPoma even though it's a neuroendocrine tumor, and we reversed the order of sucrase-isomaltase deficiency to fit the mnemonic, but you get the point!)

In **Table 1.4** we prepared a cheat sheet for IBS lookalikes to help guide you through diagnosing recalcitrant IBS. The table lists the lookalike diagnoses, clinical clues that might trigger you to consider these disorders, additional diagnostic tests to consider, and available treatments. Keep this table handy. It's solid gold.

Table 1.4. *Cheat-Sheet of IBS lookalikes.*

IBS Look-Alike	Select Clinical Clues	Diagnostic Tests	Treatments
Acute intermittent porphyria (AIP)	Intermittent pain attacks; hyponatremia; neuropathic and neuropsychiatric symptoms; dark urine; seizures; elevated transaminases	Urine PBG spot check	Hemin Givosiran
Bile acid diarrhea (BAD)	Like IBS but higher risk of incontinence; severe urgency; diarrhea in middle of the night; stool pH>6 with narrow anion gap; history of terminal ileum pathology	Fecal bile acid assay Serum C4 levels	Cholestyramine Colesevelam
Carcinoid syndrome	Explosive watery diarrhea; cutaneous flushing; bronchospasm; right-sided cardiac valve lesions; mesenteric and retroperitoneal fibrosis	Urine 5-HIAA 24h collection	Octreotide Lanreotide
Disaccharidase deficiencies (lactase; sucrase-isomaltase)	Watery diarrhea; bloating; excess gas; pain after ingesting culprit sugars; frequent and longstanding symptoms; history of physical injury or inflammation of epithelium (celiac, IBD, SIBO, AGE, giardiasis, allergic enteropathy); stool pH<6 with wide anion gap; unintentional weight loss	Small intestinal biopsy for mucosal disaccharidase assay (9% of IBS patients have SID in one study); hydrogen breath test	Diet restriction SID: sacrosidase LD: lactase
Eosinophilic gastroenteritis or colitis	Peripheral eosinophilia (usually ~80% or higher); history of allergy/atopy; protein-losing enteropathy; fat malabsorption; iron deficiency; elevated serum IgE; unintentional weight loss	Endoscopic biopsy ±full-thickness biopsy	6-food elimination diet Prednisone Budesonide
Microscopic colitis	Middle-aged; female predominant; auto-immune comorbidities; associated with certain meds (NSAIDs, PPIs); smoking	Colonic biopsy	Budesonide
Small intestinal bacterial overgrowth (SIBO)	Megaloblastic anemia with low B12 and high folate; high vit K; history of any "DYSMOTILITY" conditions (see earlier in chapter for details).	Hydrogen breath test	Antibiotics

Returning to our earlier discussion, this is where a colonoscopy could be very helpful because it might reveal underlying microscopic colitis, a condition that will not respond well to psychotherapy, tricyclic antidepressants, or other evidence-based IBS therapeutics. That's because *the patient with microscopic colitis doesn't have IBS.* We can't give up on our IBS patients if they don't respond to multiple rounds of treatment. Colonoscopy sometimes has a role to help figure things out.

We think about the INVISIBLE conditions when IBS patients don't follow the script. To be sure, we've both missed them in our own practices. Again, it is neither effective nor cost-effective to check for these conditions routinely and the ACG guidelines do not recommend you do so. But when push comes to shove and patients with IBS don't get better, then it's reasonable to look elsewhere for explanations.

Okay, so that does it for our discussion about diagnostic testing for IBS. Next, let's turn our attention to IBS treatments.

Case 1.3: Treatment of IBS-C

A 52-year-old woman presents with a longstanding history of intermittent abdominal pain and constipation that has worsened over the previous 8 months. She describes the pain as "dull and achy," usually accompanied by bloating, located in the lower abdomen, and occurring daily. She passes only 2 bowel movements per week that are usually "hard" and accompanied by excessive gas. She describes having to strain for "a couple of minutes" before spontaneously evacuating her stool, although digital disimpaction has not been necessary. She also complains of incomplete evacuation after defecation. Her abdominal pain improves with stool passage. There has been no change in stool caliber. She has no history of fevers, chills, sweats, vomiting, weight loss or rectal bleeding. She was told to eat a diet high in wheat bran and whole grains by her primary physician but complained that it caused bloating and did not improve her symptoms. She has a history of 2 normal spontaneous vaginal deliveries without complications. She has no allergies and takes no medications other than ibuprofen as needed for knee pain. She reports social alcohol use. There is no family history of gastrointestinal cancer or other significant medical conditions.

Her vital signs are normal. She has mild tenderness to palpation in the center of the abdomen. Rectal examination reveals firm stool in the vault. Her sphincter tone and perineal descent are normal. The remainder of her exam is normal.

Laboratories include a normal complete blood count, negative total IgA and anti-TTG IgA, negative fCal, and a normal CRP. A recent colonoscopy revealed scattered diverticulosis in the sigmoid colon but otherwise normal.

Know your guidelines!
1. Is further testing indicated at this time?
2. How would you treat this patient?

Case 1.3: What do the guidelines say?

Source: ACG 2021 IBS Guidelines

This is a classic case of IBS with constipation, or IBS-C. The patient meets Rome IV criteria because she has recurrent pain ≥ 1 day per week for at least the previous 3 months that is related to defecation, associated with a change in stool frequency, and associated with a change in stool form.[1] She has already received ACG guideline-recommended tests, including serologic testing for celiac disease (remember that celiac can occasionally present with constipation) and inflammatory markers in both stool and serum; they were all negative. She also received age-appropriate colonoscopy which only found scattered diverticulosis. Here's a question to ponder: does it matter that she has tics? Could that have anything to do with her IBS-C? Should it affect how you treat her? Noodle on that for a bit. We'll come back to it.

What other diagnostic tests might be warranted at this point? Well, not much. In the last vignette we discussed that testing for enteric pathogens and food allergies is not recommended here. Testing for the "INVISIBLE" diagnoses is also premature at this stage. There is also no need to conduct anorectal physiology testing since the history and physical do not reveal signs or symptoms of a pelvic floor disorder. In contrast, if she had paradoxical external anal sphincter contraction, excessive perineal descent, or other signs of anorectal dysfunction, then the ACG guidelines would suggest performing physiologic and functional testing, such as anorectal manometry or defecography. We will cover those tests later when we discuss the ACG constipation and anorectal guidelines. Bottom line here: it's time to treat.

Let's talk about IBS-C treatments. In the next vignette, we'll cover IBS-D. Some treatments can be used for both types of IBS and we'll cover those, too. Buckle up because there's a lot to discuss...

Low FODMAP Diet: Patient frequently seek advice about non-pharmacological treatments so it's important to know about the low FODMAP diet. FODMAPs are fermentable carbohydrates found in food. But not all carbohydrates are FODMAPs, just some. FODMAP is an mnemonic for:

Fermentable

Oligosaccharides

Disaccarhides

Monosaccharides

And...

Polyols

Figure 1.4A. FODMAP mnemonic.

FODMAPS ferment in the large intestine and cause GI symptoms, including bloating, cramping, abdominal pain, gas, and diarrhea. This patient does not have diarrhea, but she does have bloating, pain, and gas, so FODMAPs could still be a culprit even with IBS-C. There are 5 types of FODMAP: lactose, fructose, fructans, galacto-oligosaccharides (GOS), and polyols. **Table 1.5** lists the individual FODMAPs and common foods that contain each type.

Table 1.5. *Types of FODMAPs and foods that contain them.*

Type of FODMAP	Type of Foods
Fructans	Artichokes, asparagus, leeks, garlic, onions, wheat, chicory root, inulin
Fructose	Vegetables, sweeteners (e.g. agave, honey), fruits and fruit juices, added to processed foods and beverages (*e.g.* high-fructose corn syrup)
Galacto-oligosaccharides (GOS)	Beans (the musical fruit 😊)
Lactose	Milk, ice cream, soft cheeses (e.g. ricotta, cottage cheese), some frozen yogurts, pudding
Polyols	Fruit with pits (e.g. peaches, cherries), cauliflower, snow peas, sugar-free gum, mints and cough drops

So, does the low FODMAP diet work? Well...sort of. Let's just say it works well enough to give it a shot. The ACG guidelines recommend a *limited trial of a low FODMAP diet in patients with IBS to improve global symptoms.* A "limited trial" means 2-6 weeks; that's how long it takes to figure out if the diet is going to work. The guidelines give the diet a "conditional" recommendation and judge the quality of supporting evidence to be "very low." So, not exactly a ringing endorsement.

This is based on a meta-analysis that found the low FODMAP diet is associated with a 30% reduction in IBS symptoms compared to control diets.[26] However, the authors of that meta-analysis point out that the underlying studies are of low quality. This is an area in need of more research.

The good news is the low FODMAP diet has not been linked with serious adverse events. The notable exception is if patients remain on an over-restricted low FODMAP diet for too long, in which case it could lead to micronutrient deficiencies. For that reason, if a patient feels better on the diet, then it's important to *re-introduce* the individual FODMAPs systematically until the culprit FODMAP is identified. This is an involved process that should ideally occur in partnership with a GI dietician.

Soluble fiber: Fiber is any polymeric carbohydrate that is neither digested nor absorbed in the small intestines. Because fiber is linked to various general health benefits, and since it can interact with the gut microbiome, alter intestinal transit time, and affect stool consistency, it is commonly used as first-line therapy for IBS. But does it work? Yes…for the most part. Meta-analysis indicates that use of *soluble* fiber (found in psyllium, oat bran, barley, beans) leads to a 13% reduction in symptoms compared to control—not a huge effect, but an effect, nonetheless.[27] However, *insoluble* fiber, like the wheat bran and whole grains the patient tried in this vignette, provides *no* significant benefit for IBS symptoms. So, stick with soluble fiber when treating IBS. It's best to start low and go slow since fiber can cause bloating. The goal is to eventually work up to 25-35 grams per day. That's a lot of fiber when you consider that a single serving of psyllium powder is only 2.4 grams. Bear that in mind if someone is not responding to treatment; it might be they just don't have a large enough dose to make any difference.

Antispasmodics: Antispasmodics relax intestinal smooth muscle and reduce GI motility through a combination of direct relaxation effects, calcium channel blockade, and anticholinergic properties. The most commonly used antispasmodics for IBS are dicyclomine and hyoscyamine. Although these medications are frequently prescribed, the data supporting their efficacy is spare and low quality.[28] In addition, side effects such as dry mouth, fatigue, or worsening constipation undermine clinical benefits. For these reasons, the ACG recommends *against* using antispasmodics for IBS (admittedly, we still use them on occasion for people with urgency and cramping, not described in this vignette).

Peppermint oil: Peppermint oil has gained popularity among IBS patients because it is a natural product that is generally well tolerated. It is thought to work as calcium channel blocker with antispasmodic properties, but some theorize that peppermint oil can also modulate visceral sensitivity, has antimicrobial properties, and can even lower psychosocial distress (wow, that's a lot for a plant). Although meta-analysis of small studies reveals that peppermint oil can increase symptomatic response 2.4 times over placebo,[29] particularly for abdominal pain, a more recent study found no benefit.[30] Peppermint oil is safe and well-tolerated except for causing occasional heartburn by relaxing the lower esophageal sphincter. Overall, the guidelines support use of peppermint oil with a "conditional" recommendation.

Probiotics: This is a big topic. We don't want to dig into the probiotic literature or else we'll never quit writing. So, let's cut to the chase: the ACG guidelines recommend *against* using probiotics for IBS. The available probiotics are so different that it's challenging to study them as a group. After wading through a very complicated and heterogenous literature, the guideline authors threw up their hands and basically said *"who knows?"* We still need more high-quality studies with individual probiotic strains to figure out whether, when, and how to use them for IBS.

Fecal Transplant: Nope. Not for IBS. We'll leave it at that. More information about fecal transplant is forthcoming in G2G Volume II where we'll discuss the *C. diff* guidelines.

Polyethylene glycol (PEG) products: PEG is great for treating constipation but not great for treating IBS-C. We'll cover PEG in more detail later when we review the ACG constipation guidelines. For now, just know the IBS guidelines do *not* recommend

PEG alone for IBS since it does not improve abdominal pain, even if it does get the bowels moving. The goal with IBS is to improve both defecatory *and* sensory symptoms, not just move the bowels.

Chloride channel activators: Lubiprostone is a prostaglandin E1 analog that activates type-2 chloride channels on the intestinal epithelium. The net result is to actively pump sodium chloride into the gut lumen which passively drags bowel-softening water along with the solutes. Its clinical effect is statistically significant but rather modest, with a mean 9% symptom reduction vs placebo.[31] Diarrhea and nausea are the most common dose-limiting symptoms, with the latter occurring in up to 19% of patients in a dose-dependent manner. Since lubiprostone is generally safe and sufficiently effective, the ACG guidelines give it a "strong" recommendation.

Guanylate cyclase-C (GC-C) activators: The GC-C activators linaclotide and plecanatide both increase fluid secretion and peristalsis while reducing visceral nociception. These are useful mechanisms for IBS-C because the dual effects impact defecation (by increasing motility) *and* pain (by lowering visceral hypersensitivity). Meta-analysis shows that linaclotide reduces symptoms by 20% with an impressive number needed to treat (NNT) of 6 *vs* placebo,[32] whereas plecanatide achieves a mean 12% symptom reduction and an NNT of 9.[33] Both are well tolerated with the notable exception of diarrhea which can occasionally be dose limiting. The ACG guidelines offer a "strong" recommendation for both GC-C agonists and either one would be a great option for the patient described in this vignette.

(Are you getting tired of all these paragraphs on IBS treatment? Sorry, we did our best to grind down this massive guideline to it most salient bits, but it's a meaty one. Hang in there!)

Tricyclic antidepressants (TCAs): Both authors of this book trained at UCLA where neurogastroenterology was a prominent part of our curriculum. We learned to appreciate that IBS is not just a disorder of motility or dysbiosis but is more broadly a disorder of gut-brain interactions (DGBI). We used a lot of neuromodulators along with gut-directed psychotherapies (discussed below). We are gratified to see that, twenty years after finishing our fellowship, we were not misled. The latest IBS guidelines still "strongly" recommend use of TCAs based on extensive data supporting the efficacy and safety of these agents for improving global IBS symptoms. TCAs are especially effective for improving visceral pain and are thought to act on norepinephrine and dopaminergic receptors. As a class, TCAs reduce symptoms by 35% on average compared to placebo and confer an NNT of 4.5.[34] For this patient with IBS-C, it would be wise to select a TCA with less anticholinergic effects, such as desipramine or nortriptyline rather than amitriptyline since the latter is more constipating. The most common side effects of TCAs include dry mouth and insomnia. It's also important to ensure the QT interval is normal on EKG before starting a TCA to avoid triggering an arrhythmia.

Gut directed psychotherapies (GDPs): GDPs include cognitive behavioral therapy (CBT) and gut-directed hypnotherapy. Because IBS is a DGBI, we know that treating both poles of the brain-gut axis can improve symptoms. GDPs help patients recognize and address maladaptive cognitions, promote mindful meditation, and decrease a sense of helplessness. There is extensive evidence[35,36] supporting GDPs as an effective non-pharmacological adjunct to traditional medical therapies and the guidelines support their use.

Okay, that's it for IBS-C treatments. In the next vignette, we'll cover additional treatments that are approved for IBS-D, including rifaximin, alosetron, and eluxadoline, among others. In the meantime, **Table 1.6** summarizes the treatments we've discussed so far. The table lists each of the IBS treatments, summarizes its mechanism of action, and presents the ACG guideline recommendation and strength of evidence.

Table 1.6. *Treatments used for IBS-C.*

IBS Treatment	Mechanism of Action	ACG Recommendation	Strength of Recommendation
Low FODMAP diet	Reduce fermentable carbohydrates	Recommended	Conditional
Soluble fiber	Increase intestinal transit	Recommended	Strong
Antispasmodics	Relax intestinal smooth muscle	**Not** recommended	Conditional
Peppermint oil	Relax intestinal smooth muscle	Recommended	Conditional
Probiotics	Multiple purported mechanisms	**Not** recommended	Conditional
PEG products	Increase intestinal transit	**Not** recommended	Conditional
Chloride channel activators	Increase intestinal transit	Recommended	Strong
GC-C agonists	Increase intestinal transit, reduce visceral sensitivity	Recommended	Strong
TCAs	Reduce visceral hypersensitivity	Recommended	Strong
Gut-directed psychotherapies	CBT, GDH, mindfulness	Recommended	Conditional

But hold on a second! Remember we asked about this patient's diverticulosis? Does that impact how to treat? Maybe. There's a condition called symptomatic uncomplicated diverticular disease, or "SUDD," that looks a lot like IBS; it's basically IBS with colon tics. Although the ACG IBS guidelines do not mention SUDD, this is an important entity to know about because IBS patients with diverticulosis often ask whether the tics might be causing their symptoms. For most patients there is probably little relationship between IBS and diverticular disease. Both entities are extremely common, so it's no wonder they frequently overlap. However, for some patients the tics may trigger or propagate IBS-like symptoms. Meta-analysis indicates that using gut-directed antibiotics, like rifaximin, may be particularly useful for patients with SUDD with a very low NNT of 3.[37] It might be that tics provide tiny protective alcoves for bacteria to flourish, making antibiotics especially appealing in the management of SUDD. There is also evidence that IBS may develop after an attack of acute diverticulitis—a sort of "post-inflammatory" form of IBS rather than PI-IBS. In any event, this is a larger topic than we have room for here. See these review articles for more.[38,39]

Onward to IBS-D.

Case 1.4: Treatment of IBS-D

A 33-year-old man presents with intermittent abdominal pain and diarrhea for the past 4 years. He describes the pain as "crampy" and usually in the left lower quadrant. The pain often improves when he passes a bowel movement and is worse after eating meals. He passes 3-4 bowel movements a day that are described as "loose" and "urgent." He has no history of fevers, chills, sweats, vomiting, or rectal bleeding. There is no recent travel history, unusual food ingestions, or antibiotic use. He does not report intolerance to dairy products. He has no allergies and takes no medications.

On exam his vital signs are normal. There is mild tenderness to palpation in the left lower quadrant of the abdomen. The remainder of is examination is unremarkable.

ACG guideline-recommended tests are all negative to date, including total IgA, anti-TTG IgA, fCal, and CRP. Colonoscopy has not been performed given a lack of alarm features and young age.

The patient has already tried a low FODMAP diet in partnership with a GI dietician but did not report durable benefits. He also tried psyllium supplements at a dosage of 25g per day, but only found that it caused bloating and discomfort. Now he asks your advice for what to try next.

Know your guidelines!
1. Is further testing indicated at this time?
2. How would you treat this patient?

Case 1.4: What do the guidelines say?

Source: ACG 2021 IBS Guidelines

Just like with the patient in the last vignette, it's also too early to pursue further diagnostic testing in this IBS-D patient without alarm features. He has already received guideline-recommended testing and is otherwise too young for routine colonoscopy. Instead, it's better to move straight to treatment. If evidence-based treatments do not prove successful over time, then you can always reserve the right to conduct additional testing for the "INVISIBLE" disorders we covered earlier in the chapter. So, let's talk about some treatments specifically used for IBS-D.

Loperamide: Despite being the most widely prescribed treatment for diarrhea in North America, loperamide hardly registers in the ACG IBS guidelines except for this single line: *Loperamide is not recommended as first-line therapy for treating IBS-D symptoms because it may improve diarrhea but not improve global IBS symptoms.* And that's it for loperamide and IBS-D!

Rifaximin: As discussed earlier in this chapter, rifaximin is a non-absorbed, gut-specific antibiotic that is commonly used to treatment IBS-D. It remains unclear exactly how rifaximin works in IBS, but it is thought to modify dysbiosis found in some patients with IBS-D. Meta-analysis indicates that rifaximin has an NNT of 9 compared to placebo for reducing IBS symptoms.[40] The treatment is well tolerated and antibiotic resistance to rifaximin is extremely unusual even after multiple treatments.[41] On the basis of its safety and efficacy, the ACG guidelines offer a "strong" recommendation for use of rifaximin in IBS-D.

Alosetron: Every gastroenterologist knows the gut is our "second brain." But what does that mean? Well, lots of things. But for purpose of this discussion, it's worth noting that roughly 90% of the human body's serotonin, or 5-HT, is found in the gut, not in the brain. That's pretty crazy if you think about it. Although 5-HT modulation is often used to treat mood disorders, serotonin also has critical roles for gut function by modulating visceral sensitivity and driving motility. There are several forms of 5-HT with varying effects on GI function. A key variant is 5-HT3 which increases intestinal transit and heightens visceral sensation. As a 5-HT3 antagonist, alosetron slows intestinal transit and lowers visceral sensitivity—useful effects for IBS-D. Meta-analysis indicates that alosetron reduces IBS-D symptoms by 21% *vs* placebo and has a favorable NNT of 7.5.[42] Unfortunately, alosetron is associated with ischemic colitis and severe constipation, and on that basis it was withdrawn from the market in 2000. We remember that decision well because alosetron was widely used at the time and considered highly effective before it was unceremoniously pulled. In an unusual change of heart, the FDA reintroduced alosetron to the market after further investigation revealed a low rate of ischemic colitis (1.03 cases per 1,000 patient years of exposure) and complicated constipation (0.25 per 1,000 patient years). It is currently only approved for severe IBS-D symptoms in women who have not responded to traditional therapies.

Eluxadoline: Although opioids can slow down the bowels and lessen pain, nobody should prescribe opioids for IBS or, for that matter, most forms of visceral pain (yet opioid overuse remains too common across GI disorders[43]). However, eluxadoline offers a way to modify gut function via opioid effects without unwanted central effects. As a peripherally acting, mixed mu- and kappa-opioid receptor agonist/delta-opioid receptor antagonist (man, that's a lot of Greek letters...), eluxadoline slows intestinal transit and lowers abdominal pain without crossing the blood-brain barrier. It's fairly effective with an NNT of 10.[44] However, eluxadoline is associated with serious side effects, including acute pancreatitis in 0.4% and sphincter of Oddi spasm in 0.5%. As expected, constipation is the most common adverse event overall at 8%. Given its side effect profile, eluxadoline is contraindicated in people with a history of pancreatitis, those without a gallbladder, and those who consume more than 3 alcoholic beverages per day.

And now, finally, for the last IBS therapeutic we'll cover in this book...

Bile acid sequestrants: Earlier we discussed the "INVISIBLE" conditions that can mimic IBS. The "B" in that mnemonic stands for bile acid malabsorption, or BAM, which is caused by inadequate reabsorption of bile acids in the terminal ileum. Once bile acids enter the colon, they can trigger a secretory diarrhea and fluid losses. Although usually discussed in the context of Crohn with terminal ileal disease, BAM may also underlie some patients with IBS-D, particularly those with a history of cholecystectomy where bile delivery is misaligned with food ingestion. But even with an intact gallbladder, some patients have an idiopathic form of BAM where, for whatever reason, the terminal ileum isn't efficient at sopping up bile acids. Using the "Se-HCAT test," which is an experimental assay for BAM (not available in the U.S.), meta-analysis indicates that 28% of IBS-D patients have evidence of BAM.[45] Wow, that's a lot of BAM! (Authors peanut gallery comment: 28% seems a bit far-fetched!) Considering these results, some clinicians use bile acid sequestrants like colestipol, cholestyramine, or colesevelam to manage IBS-D. But do they work? Well, as of this writing we really don't know. The existing evidence is too sparse and too methodologically limited to make firm conclusions. That's why the ACG guidelines currently do not recommend use of bile acid sequestrants, but they ultimately conclude that *use of these therapies should be at the discretion of the clinician.*

Okay, that about does it for IBS. Let's move on to dyspepsia.

Case 1.5: Dyspepsia Management

A 54-year-old man presents with intermittent postprandial fullness, early satiety, nausea, and pain after meals for the past 12 months. He does not report heartburn. There is no history of dysphagia, vomiting, weight loss, melena, or hematochezia. He is not taking NSAIDs or aspirin and has no known history of peptic ulcer disease. Exam is unrevealing. Complete blood count is normal, electrolytes, liver tests, and screening colonoscopy are all normal.

Know your guidelines!

1. Without knowing any other information, what is the most likely underlying diagnosis?
2. What diagnostic study is warranted next?

Case 1.5: What do the guidelines say?

Source: ACG 2017 Dyspepsia Guidelines

Dyspepsia is super common. Not only that, but this pesky and burdensome symptom frequently overlaps with those of IBS, such as bloating, abdominal pain, and most every common GI symptom. We see it. *All. The. Time.*

Let's cover the dyspepsia basics, starting with a definition. The ACG dyspepsia guidelines adopt a simple and pragmatic description: *Dyspepsia is predominant epigastric pain lasting at least 1 month.* And that's it. There are separate Rome IV criteria for dyspepsia that are more complicated, but the ACG guidelines keep it simple.

Just like with IBS, *pain* is the defining feature of dyspepsia. The guidelines emphasize that dyspepsia co-occurs with other upper GI symptoms, too, including postprandial fullness, early satiety, nausea, vomiting, and heartburn. Because these symptoms are easily misunderstood, it can be useful to show pictures in clinic. **Figure 1.5** includes validated dyspepsia "pictograms" developed by Jan Tack and colleagues.[46] When the researchers used these images with patients, they found that it significantly improved communication about dyspepsia symptoms.

> Need ≥ 1 month of epigastric pain to qualify for dyspepsia

> Patients love pictures!

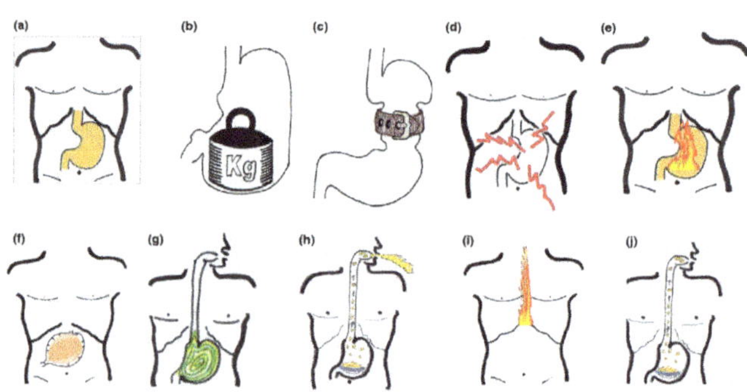

Figure 1.5. Dyspepsia pictograms to help align patient and doctor communication about common foregut symptoms. (a) location of the stomach, (b) post-prandial fullness, (c) early satiation, (d) epigastric pain, (e) epigastric burning, (f) upper abdominal bloating, (g) nausea, (h) vomiting, (i) heartburn and (j) regurgitation.[46]

No matter how you choose to communicate about dyspepsia symptoms with your patients, bear in mind that dyspepsia is not a diagnosis unto itself. It is an indication of some other underlying diagnosis. What is the most common cause of dyspepsia? Peptic ulcer disease? Esophagitis? Gallstones? *Nah!* By far and away, the most common cause of dyspepsia is functional dyspepsia (FD).

What exactly is FD? That's a big topic so we'll keep it real brief. FD is sort of like IBS of the stomach. It's defined as having dyspepsia symptoms in the setting of a normal upper endoscopy. To make things a bit more complicated, there are 2 forms of FD: epigastric pain syndrome (EPS) and postprandial distress syndrome (PDS). EPS is marked by epigastric pain or burning with eating, while PDS includes early satiety and postprandial fullness. The patient in this case most likely has EPS. In both forms of FD there are meal-related epigastric symptoms in the absence of ulcers, esophagitis, gastritis, or other organic foregut pathology.

Okay, so how to proceed? Here's what the ACG guidelines say.[47]

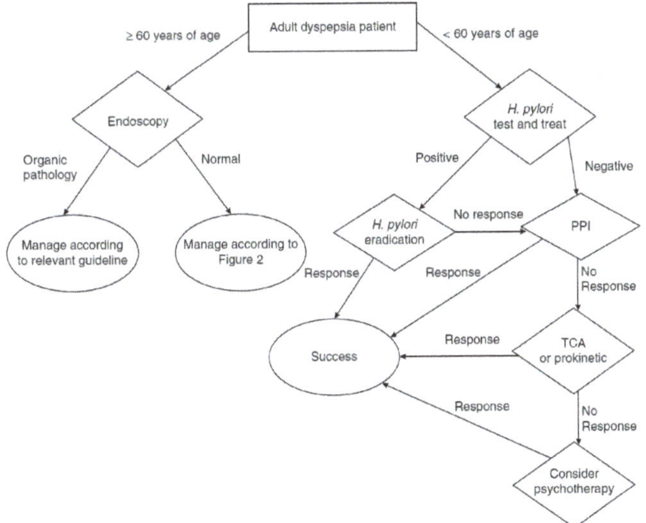

Figure 1.6. ACG dyspepsia guideline management algorithm.[47]

First, how old is your patient. Sixty or greater? Then scope 'em because you need to rule out gastric cancer. If the scope is normal, then the diagnosis is FD and you manage them accordingly (more on that shortly).

If your patient is less than 60 years old, as with this case, then endoscopy is not warranted. The next step is to test for *H. pylori* and treat the infection if positive. We'll cover the details of *H. pylori* treatment in Volume II of the G2G series.

If your patient is negative for *H. pylori*, then the next step is to administer an empirical trial of proton pump inhibitor (PPI) therapy and monitor for response. If there's no benefit, then proceed to a trial of TCAs or a prokinetic. If those treatments do not work, then next up is to "consider psychotherapy." Note that this sequence repeats if your patient is over 60 years of age and has a negative endoscopy, also suggesting a diagnosis of FD (**Figure 1.6** refers to "Figure 2" from the guidelines, not reproduced here because it's the same PPI→TCA/prokinetic→psychotherapy sequence we just discussed).

According to the algorithm, all options eventually lead to "success" (see **Figure 1.6**). If only that were true in real life! Unfortunately, we're not living in a fantasy world where all roads lead to the treasure chest. Like with all guidelines, there's only so far the document can go before devolving into a patient-by-patient decision aid. So, we get it: the guideline can't cover every possible situation. Realistically, if a patient fails to respond to the sequence shown in **Figure 1.6**, then it's time to try out other stuff not discussed in the guideline, like...a lot of stuff. Everything from virtual reality (VR) treatment,[48] to pregabalin,[49] to mirtazapine,[50] to, well, you get the point. It's your call and the guidelines do not go into detail on how to proceed if you fail to reach the "success" circle.

Oh, right, what about the situation where your patient is under 60 years old but has alarm features, like unintended weight loss, dysphagia, or anemia? Shouldn't they be scoped? You might think so. But the ACG guidelines say no, they *shouldn't* necessarily be scoped. The reason is that alarm features are not terribly sensitive and specific for cancer. In addition, the guidelines emphasize that gastric cancer remains a rare cause of dyspepsia in younger North American patients. That said, we readily acknowledge that every case should be considered on its own merits and sometimes an endoscopy is warranted even if the guidelines say otherwise. The guidelines also indicate that age thresholds are not immutable and that alarm features, although not as important as other guidelines indicated in the past, should certainly not be ignored.

Case 1.6: Management of Defecatory Disorders

A 63-year-old woman presents with problems with constipation for the past 4 decades. She describes straining on the commode to eventually release "bunny pellets" after using suppositories and digital maneuvering in her anus or vagina. She has been eating whole grains, beans, figs, prunes, and leafy vegetables at every meal. Furthermore, she has supplemented a high fiber diet with psyllium, drinks plenty of water and exercises twice daily to no avail. Stimulant laxatives minimally improve her sensation of incomplete fecal evacuation. There have been no alarm signs or symptoms and there has been no history of rectal trauma or instrumentation. She states that she had a negative screening colonoscopy earlier this year at another GI practice. Due to the persistence of her symptoms, she has remained frustrated and now seeks your expert guidance.

On anorectal exam you note that perineal descent exceeds 3 cm while bearing down. There is a non-tender and soft external hemorrhoid. Digital rectal examination does not reveal paradoxical contraction of the external anal sphincter during simulated defecation. There is a hardened ball of stool which inhibits your ability to further examine the anatomy of the rectal vault. There is no evidence of blood or obvious masses. The remainder of her physical examination is unremarkable.

Know your guidelines!
1. What is the next diagnostic step?
2. What treatment should you offer this patient?

Case 1.6: What do the guidelines say?

Source: ACG 2021 Management of Benign Anorectal Disorders Guidelines

We'll get to the answer in a moment. But first, have you ever seen a hemorrhoid in your practice? Are any of your patients constipated? What about painful defecation? Ever seen that?

Ummm…yeah, like every day of the week!

Among the 70+ guidelines published by the ACG, the document on benign anorectal disorders might be the most widely applicable to everyday general GI practice. Even if you're a hepatologist, interventional endoscopist, IBDologist, or a pseudoxanthoma elasticologist, you undoubtedly encounter hemorrhoids, fissures, incontinence, fecal impaction, and other benign anorectal disorders most every day. If you take care of humans in your clinical practice, then this guideline is for you.

Okay, this patient has constipation, sure, but it's not an ordinary case of constipation. She has features that suggest a defecatory disorder (DD). DDs are defined as difficulty evacuating stool from the rectum in patients with constipation.[51] Diagnosing a DD requires formal evidence of disrupted evacuation on functional testing, which we'll discuss shortly.

But first, let's consider what it takes to push out a bowel movement. Think of it like squeezing toothpaste out of a tube. Three things are required to get out the paste: (1) you've got to squeeze the tube; (2) you've got to direct the squeeze towards the cap; and (3) you've gotta remove the cap.[52] If any of those steps goes wrong, well, then you won't be brushing your teeth. **Figure 1.7** shows the 3 mechanisms and lists example DDs where each mechanism goes awry.

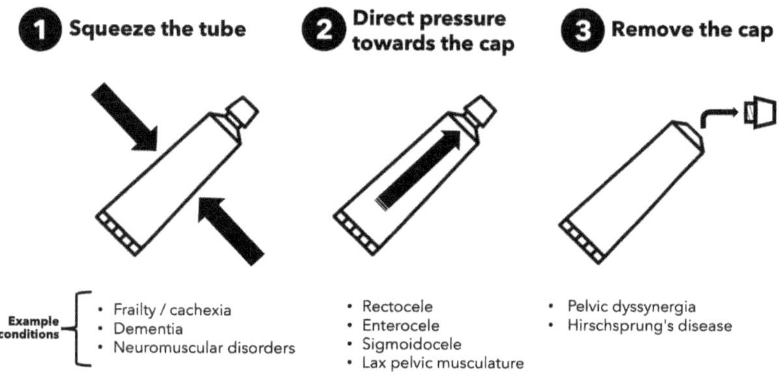

Figure 1.7. Three steps to squeezing out toothpaste, with analogous DDs.

Stuff can go wrong with each of these steps. For example, frail patients with cachexia, dementia, or neuromuscular disorders might be unable to contract their abdomen with sufficient force to expel stool from the rectum. These patients cannot squeeze the tube, so the toothpaste stays put.

For others, there may be plenty of squeeze power, but the pressure wave moves in the wrong direction. Those with a rectocele, as should be suspected in this patient case, will push stool into a blind pouch and divert flow away from the anus. Those with lax pelvic musculature and/or a rectocele may also experience excessive perineal descent and struggle to push stool out the chute.

Others may have plenty of squeeze pressure directed towards the exit, but the exit is blocked. What would do that? For one, the tube needs to be straight. If you've got a kink in the tube, then the toothpaste will back up. That's what happens when the puborectalis sling—that angle-forming ring around the rectum that maintains continence—fails to relax during defecation. Same thing if you don't relax your external anal sphincter; that's like keeping the cap on the tube. No good. In rare circumstances there may be residual short segment Hirschsprung's disease that persists undetected into adulthood. In that case there is lack of reflex inhibition of the internal anal sphincter due to lack of enteric inhibitor neurons, leading to outlet obstruction.

In all cases you'll get the same result: pooping problems.

How can you tell whether someone with constipation has a DD rather than a more proximal cause of constipation, like slow-transit constipation? Start by listening for a story of excessive straining, a sense of anorectal blockage, perception of incomplete evacuation, need for manual maneuvers (i.e., inserting a finger into the anus or pushing posteriorly from within the vagina, as described in this vignette), or a story of protruding tissue during defecation (which might indicate rectal prolapse). Just bear in mind that these symptoms, unto themselves, do not distinguish between a DD and other forms of constipation.[53] More testing will be required to clinch the diagnosis.

How do you diagnose a DD? *Start with your finger.* Performing a digital rectal examination (DRE) has become a lost art. We don't mean to sound like grumpy old professors here, but too few residents, fellows, and GI practitioners perform a DRE anymore. And we mean *any* DRE, not even a complete DRE. Just no DRE at all. We (and others[54]) have even seen an occasional GI colleague skip the DRE using the excuse that a colonoscopy is planned, so why inconvenience the patient? Well, assuming your patient is willing to be examined and there is an available chaperone, then there are 2 contraindications to DRE in non-neutropenic patients with DD symptoms: either you do not have a finger, or the patient does not have a rectum!*

As we were putting the finishing touches on this book, one of your authors got an inpatient consult for lower abdominal pain and constipation. This patient had been examined by no fewer than 5

---

* We credit the late, great, Fred Weinstein, MD, our former fellowship program director and GI extraordinaire, with first teaching us these two contraindications.

doctors on the inpatient wards before we were called to sort things out. On history, the patient explained that she had "tissue" coming out of her anus that she had to push back in. Had a rectal exam been documented? No. Not at all. So, we took a look. And literally, all we had to do was look; no finger required. We simply asked her to bear down and, voila, her rectum prolapsed straight out her anus. It was unmissable, but everyone had missed it. Not cool.

So, you guessed it, this patient needs a DRE. The ACG guidelines describe how to perform a DRE and we'll assume that you already know the basics. In short, a complete DRE can identify anal fissures, hemorrhoids, fecal impaction, rectal prolapse and descending perineum syndrome (consider when perineal descent exceeds 3 cm on Valsalva maneuver). You can also diagnose dyssynergic defecation with 75% sensitivity and 87% specificity compared to anorectal manometry[55] (feel for paradoxical sphincter contraction during simulated defecation, which is not evident in this case). Beyond that, a full DRE allows you to palpate the puborectalis sling and monitor its contractility during evacuation, establish baseline anal sphincter tone, estimate squeeze pressure, and determine the anorectal angle at rest and during defecation. You can also feel for presence of a stool ball that might lead to both constipation and overflow incontinence. As an aside, if fecal impaction is suspected but not detected by DRE, then consider doing a KUB to rule out higher impaction. In any event, that's a lot of info from one finger! The DRE accomplishes way more than just checking for 'rhoids and feeling for masses. Your index finger is a full-on diagnostic machine!

This patient most likely has a rectocele, although you can't know for sure without further examination and testing. On DRE, a rectocele may be detected by feeling your finger dip into an indentation along the anterior rectal wall when the patient bears down. It can be more obvious if there's a concurrent protrusion through the vagina, which likely explains why this patient needed to splint her vagina to ease defecation. That was hard to detect here because a stool ball filled the rectal vault, impeding a full anatomic examination.

The vagina and rectum are 2 muscular tubes that share a common wall known as the rectovaginal septum separating the posterior vagina and anterior rectum. When this common wall becomes weak, which can especially occur in women who have vaginal deliveries, then a rectocele may form. **Figure 1.8** shows this anatomic relationship and likely explains why the patient in this vignette needed to insert a finger into the vagina to facilitate stool passage.

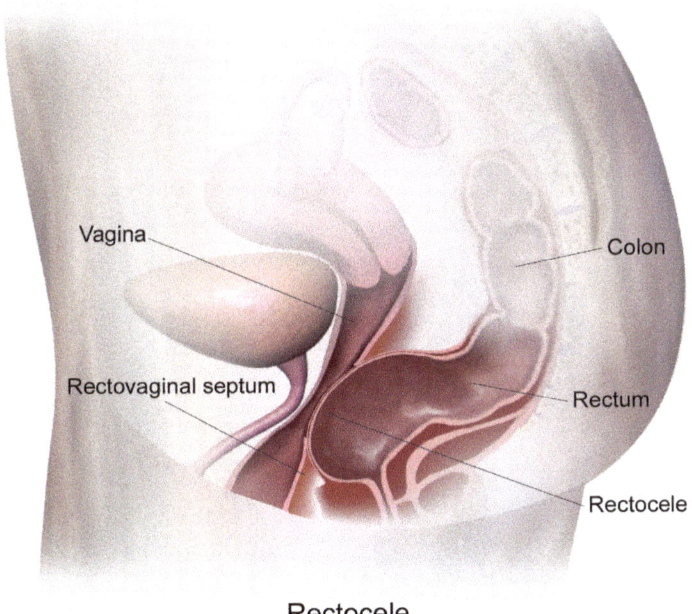

Figure 1.8. Anatomic relationship between the rectum, vagina, and a rectocele. Image used under creative commons license from Wikimedia commons.

Okay, so you should suspect a rectocele in this patient. Her DRE does not suggest pelvic dyssynergia, but it does reveal excessive perineal descent which could mean there's a rectocele, lax pelvic musculature, or some other structural issue. It's hard to know at this stage without further testing. What to do next? The ACG guidelines provide the algorithm shown in **Figure 1.9.**

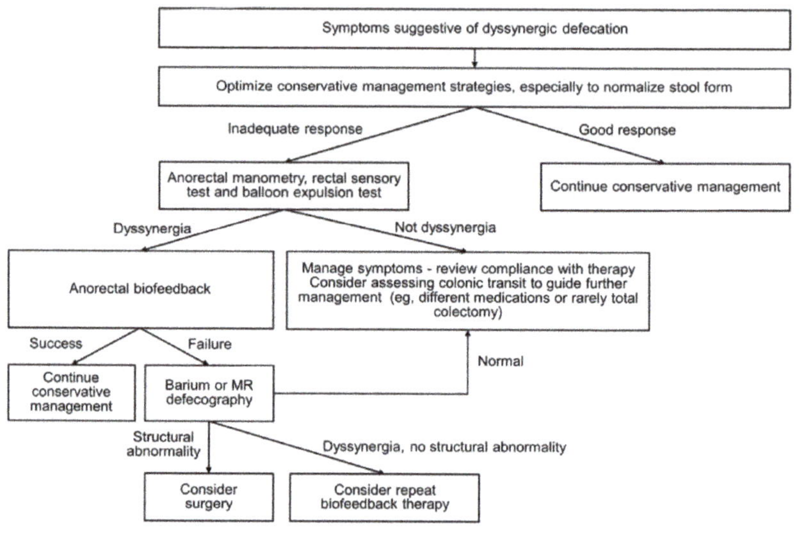

Figure 1.9. ACG algorithm for managing patients with a possible DD.

Suspect a DD? Conservative management comes before testing

The first step is to optimize conservative management focused on normalizing stool form. This includes using fiber supplement or laxatives, considering a footstool to enhance defecation by opening the anorectal angle (we love a good footstool!), and advising to eat meals of 500 kcal or greater to trigger the gastrocolic reflex. Although not mentioned in the guidelines, a randomized controlled trial also found that self-performed perineal massage can break up stool in the rectal vault and enhance defection.[56] Seriously. It can really work for the motivated patient. Other recommendations include pooping when nature calls (i.e., don't hold it in), avoiding straining during defecation, and avoiding lengthy bathroom sessions. For more on the general management of constipation, check out our discussion on the ACG constipation guidelines later in this chapter.

Table 1.7. *Conservative treatment strategies for DDs.*

Try a soluble fiber supplement
Consider a laxative
Use a footstool during defecation
Massage that perineum (carefully)
Eat 500 kcal meals to kick-start the gastrocolic reflex
Don't hold your poop
Try not to strain
Limit time sitting on the toilet

Now, if conservative therapy works, then great. But if it doesn't, then it's time for formal testing. The guidelines describe a list of tests that we won't review in detail here. In short, the next step is to perform both an anorectal manometry (ARM) *and* a balloon expulsion test (BET) using a standard 50cc balloon. Not just one test. Not just the other test. But *both tests*.

Why perform both an ARM and a BET? The reason is that false-positive and false-negative results can occur with either test alone, so performing them together improves diagnostic accuracy. Separately, the Rome IV guidelines also require 2 abnormal tests to diagnose a DD.[57] Of note, some people might jump to a defecography at this stage, but the ACG guidelines recommend holding on defecography until later in the algorithm, if needed, since it is more expensive, cumbersome, and, in the case of barium defecography, requires radiation. Our caveat is this: if you had a patient like the one in this vignette with excessive perineal descent but no signs of dyssynergia on DRE, and if the ARM were normal but the BET were abnormal, then it might still be extremely useful to obtain a defecography sooner than later. In that instance, the normal ARM and DRE would argue against a dyssynergic pattern, but the abnormal BET would still indicate

Conservative management fails for DD symptoms? Do ARM and BET together next

ARM negative but BET positive? Might now be dyssynergia, but could still be a structural issue like a rectocele that something is impacting evacuation. Assuming the patient can exert enough abdominal pressure (mechanism #1 in **Figure 1.7**) and knowing that they don't have an outlet problem (mechanism #3), then it suggests there's a structural problem with the rectum or pelvic floor, like a rectocele or lax pelvic musculature (mechanism #2). That's where the defecography is most useful.

If the ARM and BET reveal dyssynergia, meaning inappropriate contraction of the external anal sphincter and/or puborectalis during defecation, then you should initiate anorectal biofeedback.

The details of biofeedback are beyond what we will cover here; check out the guidelines to learn more. In short, biofeedback teaches patients how to perform abdominal breathing, instructs on how to generate sufficient force to evacuate their rectum, and teaches patients how to loosen their sphincter during defecation. It literally teaches people how to be less anal retentive. The guidelines recommend 4 to 6 sessions, each several weeks apart, to achieve full therapeutic benefits.

Anorectal manometry usually works very well. But what if it doesn't? What then? The answer is defecography. Assuming you haven't already ordered this test (because, say, you strongly suspected a rectocele early on), then you would order it once the patient

fails anorectal biofeedback because there might be a structural issue that's gone undetected. There are 2 forms of defecography: magnetic resonance (MR) and barium defecography. Most centers use barium since it's simpler, cheaper, and can be performed in the seated position, thereby mimicking defecation. In contrast, MR defecography must be performed with the patient on their side. But MR is better at measuring pelvic floor motion and detecting organ prolapse and it doesn't require radiation. The choice between barium and MR comes down to local preference and expertise.

If the defecography reveals a sizeable (*i.e.,* 5 cm), non-emptying rectocele or significant rectal prolapse, then these conditions may be effectively treated with surgery and conservative measures are likely to fail. Same thing if you find a sigmoidocele or enterocele. The details of surgery are beyond this discussion. Assuming you have excluded any co-existing defecatory disorders beyond the rectocele, refer these patients to colorectal surgery for further evaluation.

Case 1.7: Management of Fecal Incontinence

A 68-year-old man with a history of medically controlled hypertension, benign prostatic hypertrophy, and osteoarthritis presents with a chief complaint of fecal incontinence. He describes feeling an urge to defecate and often rushes to the bathroom but cannot make it in time before soiling himself. He experiences 2-3 episodes of fecal incontinence per week for the past 8 months. He describes loose and watery stools that are non-bloody. He does not have abdominal pain, unintended weight loss or other alarm symptoms. There is no known history of ulcerative proctitis and no history of prostate cancer or pelvic radiation. The patient denies any history of rectal trauma or instrumentation. He does not report urinary incontinence or erectile dysfunction. His medications include lisinopril, ibuprofen, and finasteride. He comes to you with previous workup including a normal complete blood count and metabolic panel, normal fecal calprotectin, normal CRP, and a normal screening colonoscopy from 4 years ago. His primary care physician ordered labs for enteric pathogens that were normal. He has not received recent antibiotics.

Prior to seeing you, he was treated conservatively with loperamide and pelvic floor exercises. He also received education about fecal incontinence. However, his symptoms persisted despite these initial steps. He is sent to you for further examination and work-up.

Digital rectal exam now reveals an intact anal wink on pinprick testing but weak external anal sphincter squeeze pressure. There is no stool in the vault, no masses, and normal amount of perineal descent when bearing down. The remainder of his physical examination is unremarkable.

Know your guidelines!

What is the next step in the diagnostic work-up for this patient's fecal incontinence?

Case 1.7: What do the guidelines say?

Source: ACG 2021 Management of Benign Anorectal Disorders Guidelines

Fecal incontinence (FI) is more common than many people realize. Population-based surveys reveal an overall age-adjusted FI prevalence of 9% in the US,[58] with up to 50% of nursing home residents experiencing this disabling symptom.[59] That means you probably see a lot of FI in your practice. It also means you should ask about FI routinely because many people have it, yet few proactively discuss FI due to fear, stigma, or shame around their incontinence. **Table 1.8** lists risk factors and medical conditions associated with FI that should trigger you to inquire about this symptom.

Table 1.8. *Risk factors and medical conditions associated with FI.*

Older age
Female
History of diarrhea
Fecal impaction (overflow incontinence)
Urinary incontinence (marker of sacral nerve injury)
Obstetric anal sphincter injury
Diabetic neuropathy
Spinal cord injury
Proctitis (e.g., from inflammatory bowel disease)

There are 2 general categories of FI: *urge incontinence* and *passive incontinence.* The difference comes down to whether the patient is aware of the need to defecate before stooling occurs. If a patient feels a strong urge to defecate but cannot make it to the bathroom in time, as in this case, then we call it urge incontinence. On the other hand, if stool leaks from the anus without forewarning, then it's passive incontinence.

The mechanisms of urge incontinence and passive incontinence are different albeit sometimes overlapping. **Figure 1.10** outlines the various mechanisms of FI. Patients with urge incontinence often have diminished squeeze pressure and duration, which is governed by the external anal sphincter (EAS). In contrast, those with passive incontinence have diminished resting pressure, which is maintained by the internal anal sphincter (IAS). That's a key difference. Whereas the EAS is under voluntary control and is formed of striated muscle, the IAS is under autonomic—not voluntary—control and is made of smooth muscle. Thus, conditions that affect the autonomic nervous system, such as diabetes, may affect the IAS. In contrast, the EAS is typically affected by mechanical trauma, such as from childbirth, or through damage to the pudendal nerve, which carries somatic (not autonomic) fibers to the EAS. In addition, if the rectum is inflamed, as with ulcerative proctitis, then it becomes hypersensitive and wants to jettison contents quickly. In other cases, there might be diminished rectal capacity or low distensibility, as with radiation proctopathy. Another trigger of incontinence is severe constipation with fecal impaction; this can lead to anal seepage of stool and often presents with passive "overflow" incontinence and soiling of undergarments. **Figure 1.10** summarizes these mechanisms of FI.

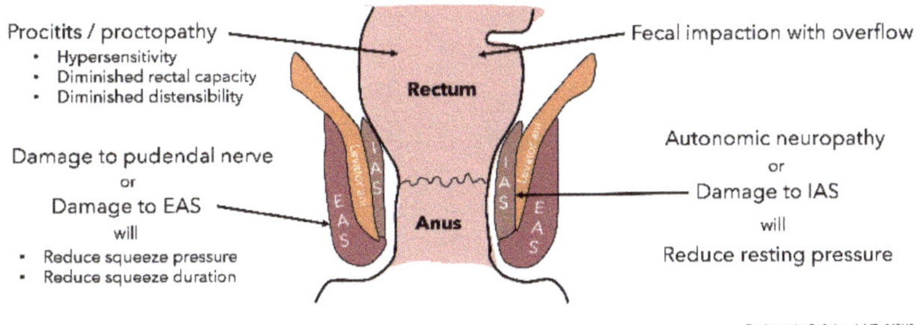

Figure 1.10. Mechanisms of urge incontinence and passive incontinence. The mechanisms are not mutually exclusive; multiple causes of FI may co-exist in the same patient. While we're here, a side note: the levator ani muscle sits between the IAS and EAS. It can sometimes become strained or tensed, leading to severe anorectal pain. This is called "levator ani syndrome" and ACG guidelines suggest treating it with biofeedback if there's evidence of dyssynergic defecation on ARM.

Just like with DDs, evaluating FI also mandates performing a careful DRE. Beyond the numerous DRE assessments we discussed in the last case (look back for the details), here you should also perform perianal pinprick testing. Although traditionally performed with an actual pin, you can just break a wooden tongue depressor and use its sharp edge to perform this test. Lightly prick the edge of the anal sphincter and then watch for the reflex anal "wink" (a rather descriptive term). This procedure measures the integrity of the sacral lower motor neuron reflex arc and is an important screen for sacral root compression or other spinal injuries. If there is no anal wink, then the test is "positive" and you should investigate further. Remember that S2, S3, and S4 govern the "*3Ps*"—*p*ooping, *p*eeing, and *p*enile erections—so ask about concurrent urinary incontinence and, in men, erectile dysfunction. If there is any concern about a spinal injury, then you should consider ordering a lumbosacral MRI and/or conferring with a neurosurgeon or neurologist. Beyond the pinprick test, check the EAS squeeze pressure, feel for a stool ball in the rectum, assess IAS resting pressure, and while you're at it, inspect the undergarments

> Do a pinprick test for all patients with FI. If positive, consider spinal MRI

for evidence of soilage. There's so much you can do with the DRE, so don't skip it!

Assuming there is no sign of spinal injury and the patient's symptoms are otherwise manageable, then conservative treatment is warranted. The ACG guidelines list 3 components to initial treatment: (1) education about the potential causes of FI for each patient (this should be individualized); (2) if there is concurrent diarrhea, then slow down the bowels with loperamide or diphenoxylate along with soluble fiber supplements; and (3) teach pelvic floor exercises to strengthen the pelvic floor musculature. Although not listed among the 3 pillars of conservative therapy, patients with suspected overflow incontinence and fecal impaction should be treated for constipation; just monitor closely to make sure symptoms do not worsen.

If conservative therapy fails, as occurred in this case, then the next step is more advanced diagnostic testing with ARM, rectal BET, and rectal sensation testing. These tests should ideally be performed in a motility lab with ample experience performing and interpreting these sophisticated exams. We will skip the details here; check out the ACG guidelines and other resources, such as guidance published by the American Neurogastroenterology and Motility Society (ANMS),[60] for details on how to perform and analyze these tests in an FI patient.

The next step depends on what's found during specialized anorectal testing. If there is diminished squeeze pressure or low resting tone, for example, then endoanal ultrasound and/or MRI may be warranted to look for a sphincter tear or disruption; this might respond well to surgery and should be evaluated by an experienced colorectal surgeon. If there is no structural damage or evidence of spinal root injury (*e.g.,* on needle EMG of the anal sphincter), then anorectal biofeedback is warranted. Again, we'll leave the details of FI biofeedback training to the guidelines for those interested in learning more.

What should you do if biofeedback therapy fails? There are a few remaining options. One is to use an anal plug as a mechanical barrier device. Data indicate that around 60% of people find the plug to be helpful.[61] Another approach for women with refractory FI is to use an intravaginal balloon. When fitted correctly (which is not always easy), the balloon compresses the anterior rectal wall and serves as a mechanical barrier. In one study the balloon helped reduce FI symptoms in 86% of users.[62] A less fancy approach is just to use cotton balls in the anus to help absorb smaller amounts of anal seepage. Yet another option is to inject an FDA-cleared bulking agent into the anal sphincter. When using dextranomer in hyaluronic acid, injection therapy improves symptoms in around half of recipients and outperforms placebo injections.[63]

In severe cases that do not respond to mechanical barrier treatments, some turn to sacral nerve stimulation (SNS) or, in the most recalcitrant cases, colostomy with an end stoma. But these should be reserved for patients with uncontrolled symptoms despite biofeedback and barrier treatments.

Case 1.8: Management of Gastroparesis

A 31-year-old woman with a long history of chronic constipation presents to the clinic with 5 months of postprandial fullness, bloating with lower abdominal pain accompanied with vomiting several times per week. She states that she sleeps well without nocturnal symptoms. However, she has lost 8 pounds since these symptoms started over the past 5 months. She has no prior surgeries and no other medical problems. She takes no medications, narcotics, cannabinoids, or herbals. Physical examination is unremarkable. You note that the following studies were normal at her primary care provider's office: CBC, CMP, lipase, TSH, hemoglobin A1c, abdominal ultrasound.

Know your guidelines!

1. What is the next diagnostic step?
2. What is the first treatment that you should offer?

Case 1.8: What do the guidelines say?

Source: ACG 2022 Management of Gastroparesis Guidelines

Earlier in this chapter we covered dyspepsia, a common condition that GI docs see most every day of the week. But sometimes what seems like a simple case of dyspepsia might actually be gastroparesis (GP) lurking under the surface. As we'll see in this chapter, there is a spectrum between GP and functional dyspepsia (FD) and the 2 conditions can be easily confused. So, how can you tell when a patient with meal-related foregut symptoms has GP? And what is GP, anyway? The ACG guidelines offer this definition:

> *GP is a motility disorder characterized by symptoms and objective documentation of delayed gastric emptying of solid food without mechanical obstruction, which should be excluded by imaging studies such as upper GI endoscopy or radiology. The chronic symptoms experienced by patients with GP may be associated with acute exacerbation of symptoms after oral intake of food; the symptoms include post-prandial fullness, nausea, vomiting, and upper abdominal pain.*[64]

This definition has a few important components. First, remember that GP symptoms are related to solid food ingestion, not just liquid ingestion. If symptoms occur immediately after sipping some water, for example, then that may not be GP. But if post-prandial fullness and other cardinal GP symptoms occur after eating solid food, then GP is in the differential. Also, since GP is meal related, it would be unusual for symptoms to show up randomly in the middle of the night or to frequently arise when fasting. Of course, FD-symptoms are *also* meal related, so this feature alone does not distinguish GP from FD. Second, you cannot make a diagnosis of GP without foregut imaging, just as you cannot diagnose FD without an upper endoscopy. Third, there is considerable symptom overlap between FD and GP since both can cause post-prandial fullness, upper abdominal pain, and nausea.

However, it is rare for FD to cause frequent vomiting. The patient in this vignette is vomiting several times per week after eating, which is less consistent with FD and instead suggests delayed gastric emptying either from a motility disorder or, possibly, from a partial gastric outlet obstruction. You can't tell those apart without endoscopy or imaging.

This patient also has constipation and bloating, which might make you think about IBS or SIBO. It is possible that she has a few syndromes at once. Keep in mind that the human body doesn't draw a dotted line at the pylorus to cordon-off the stomach from the rest of the GI tract. It's not like the body has memorized the Rome criteria or aligned neatly with textbook chapters. In fact, many patients with GP also have dysmotility elsewhere in their gut—not just in the stomach—and may suffer from both small bowel and colonic dysmotility. When a patient with foregut symptoms also has bloating, constipation, and other gut symptoms, think about a more diffuse dysmotility pattern that might accompany delayed gastric emptying. If the stomach is slow, then the rest of the GI tract may be slow, too.

Oh, by the way, you'll notice in the definition of GP that abdominal pain is a common symptom. Most people think of postprandial fullness, nausea, and vomiting when they think of GP, but not everyone thinks about pain. However, up to 90% of people with GP in referral centers have abdominal pain.[65] Moreover, although upper abdominal pain is common, the pain might also be perceived as mid- or even lower-abdominal as seen with this patient. Remember that GP frequently presents with diffuse abdominal pain, not just classic dysmotility-type symptoms.

There are many risk factors for GP. It is helpful to group GP as idiopathic (the most common at 40%-50% of cases), diabetic (~30%), iatrogenic (e.g., from surgery or medications), or related to another non-diabetic disorder. If a patient develops GP symptoms after starting an opioid or other culprit medication, like an anticholinergic, GLP-1 agonist, or dopamine agonist, then consider iatrogenic GP and stop the medication whenever possible before launching into a diagnostic workup. If there is a history of vagotomy or fundoplication, then you should also think about iatrogenic GP from surgery. In other cases, GP might be an early sign of a neurodegenerative condition like Parkinson's disease, or multiple sclerosis. It may also accompany connective tissue disorders like systemic sclerosis and lupus. Or you might see it with vascular disorders, hypothyroidism, adrenal insufficiency, or hypopituitarism. Note that marijuana can also delay gastric emptying. When a patient is not diabetic, has no history of vagotomy, is not on the usual culprit meds or substances, and does not have an obvious culprit disorder, then you're in the common territory of idiopathic GP. These cases are often caused by post-viral dysmotility from previous infection with HSV, CMV, and VZV. That's a lot of GP risk factors to remember, so we made (yet another) mnemonic to help you memorize the full list. Check out **Figure 1.11**.

G astric surgery / GLP-1 agonists

A myloidosis / Anticholinergics / Adrenal insufficiency

S ystemic sclerosis

T hyroid disease / THC

R adiation injury

O pioids

P arkinson's / Pancreatitis

A lzheimer's

R heumatic & connective tissue disorders

E ndocrinopathies (especially <u>diabetes</u>)

S hy-Drager syndrome

I <u>diopathic</u> / infections

S ystemic illness (e.g., from severe renal, liver, or vascular disease)

Figure 1.11. The risk factors and causes of GP conveniently spell out GASTROPARESIS! (We were very excited when we figured this out). Underlined conditions are most common, with idiopathic at #1 (40-50% of cases) and diabetes at #2 (~30%).

The patient in this vignette does not have diabetes, a vagotomy, or a known history of neurodegenerative or connective tissue disorders. She is not taking any culprit medications or cannabinoids. You should suspect GP because she has recurrent meal related symptoms including nausea, vomiting, postprandial fullness, and abdominal pain. She is losing weight, too, which is concerning for nutritional deficiencies. She also describes bloating and constipation which may occur with GP. **Figure 1.12** displays the ACG algorithm for how to proceed[64].

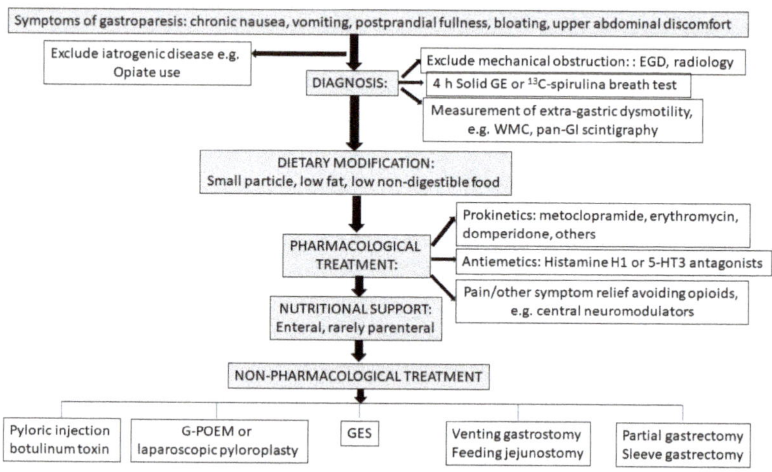

Figure 1.12. ACG algorithm for the diagnosis and management of GP. GE, gastric emptying; GES, gastric electrical stimulation; G-POEM, gastric per-oral endoscopic myotomy; WMC, wireless motility capsule.[64]

Start with an upper endoscopy to rule-out a mechanical outlet obstruction, such as gastric cancer, a bezoar, or a pyloric channel ulcer with an edematous and obstructed outflow tract. While you're in there, look for indirect evidence of gastric dysmotility, such as bile reflux gastropathy and/or excessive pooling of gastric contents or retained food. Just be aware that these findings are not sensitive or specific for GP and should not be used as a substitute for definitive testing.

Endoscopic evidence of GP is insufficient to make the diagnosis

Once you have ruled-out a mechanical obstruction, the next step is to document the presence of delayed gastric emptying. The most definitive test is a scintigraphic gastric emptying (SGE) study, but the 13-carbon spirulina breath test is another acceptable option. Let's talk about these tests.

SGE Study: Most people use the SGE test to diagnose GP because it's considered the gold standard. Be sure to stop any medications or substances that affect gastric motility at least 48 hours before the test, including opioids, cannabinoids, prokinetics, antiemetics, and neuromodulators. Also be sure that glucose is well-controlled prior to the test. The SGE involves eating a 2% low-fat eggbeater meal that is radiolabeled and monitored over a minimum of 3 hours, and ideally *4 hours*. This is key: if the SGE is performed for less than 3 hours, then it may lead to false positive results.[66] For some reason, many labs still only perform a 90-minute exam and then claim the test is positive if too much food is retained, but it's within normal limits to retain food after 90 minutes. You've got to wait longer than that. During the SGE test, scans need only be obtained once per hour, not every 10 minutes as performed in the past; there is no extra benefit of scanning that often.[67] If more than 10% of the meal is retained in the stomach after 4 hours (i.e., $\leq$90% emptying), then the test is positive for GP. Sometimes you'll find a mild delay in emptying that does not meet GP criteria but may suggest FD if there are typical foregut symptoms. You can appreciate there's a spectrum between GP and FD with the former exhibiting more pronounced dysmotility than the latter.[68] Truth be told, the 10% SGE retention rule is a bit arbitrary and some centers still use the 20% cut-off, but we need to draw the line somewhere.

13-Carbon Spirulina Study: This is an FDA-approved, commercially available, easily administered breath test that can be performed in an office setting. Patient consume a scrambled egg mix containing ^{13}C-spirulina which is absorbed in the upper small intestine. Then, the patient provides periodic breath samples into tubes which are sent to a centralized lab and tested for presence of $^{13}CO2$. The test has been validated against the SGE study and is considered an acceptable, less invasive, non-radioactive alternative to the SGE.[69] The ACG guidelines refer to the breath test as "reliable" and recommend it as a viable option.

Let's say either the SGE or breath test comes back positive. What next? **Figure 1.12** shows that dietary modification is the first therapeutic step before starting any meds. So, let's talk diet.

A quick word about the GP diet: The most important thing about the GP diet is that food should be consumed as small particles. Randomized controlled trial data indicate that a small-particle diet is superior to a large particle diet, so patients should be instructed to eat foods with the consistency of mashed potatoes.[70] If needed, they should blend their food to reach a mashed potato consistency so it can easily pass through the pylorus, which requires a diameter of 2mm or less (that's small!). Anything with husks, peels, membranes, seeds, or crunchy grains should be minimized or avoided when possible. That includes the foods listed in **Table 1.9**, below. It's also good to avoid fatty foods and foods with high non-digestible fiber which might slow gastric emptying time.

Table 1.9. *Example foods to minimize in a GP diet.*

Food with Husks/Peels	Foods with membranes	Stringy foods	Seeds and grains	Poorly digestible food
Corn	Orange	Rhubarb	Nuts	Rice
Peas	Lemons	Asparagus	Almonds	Raw vegetables
Tomato	Grapefruit	Leeks	Bread with	Meat
Sprouts		Stalks of	whole grain	Cheese slices
Onions		broccoli		
Cabbage		Cauliflower		

If diet manipulation does not provide sufficient relief, then the next step is to consider medical treatments for refractory GP. There are 2 mechanistic goals of medical therapy: increase gastric emptying and decrease nausea and vomiting. Some meds work on motility but do little for nausea, whereas others only address nausea but do not promote gastric motility. Some do both. Thus, it's important to ask patients about their most bothersome symptom: is it in the nausea/vomiting category or the postprandial fullness/discomfort category? The answer might determine whether you use a promotility agent, antiemetic agent, or both. It's also important to know that the correlation between gastric emptying time and GP symptoms is tenuous, raising questions about whether GP is really a pure motor problem, a sensory problem, or both. Unfortunately, promoting gastric motility alone does not always improve GP symptoms, but we often try it anyway and hope for the best because our options remain limited for refractory GP. Here are the key meds to know about from the ACG guidelines:

> Speeding up gastric emptying does not necessarily improve GP symptoms (unfortunately)

Metoclopramide: Love it or hate it, we're still stuck with metoclopramide. Although some shy away from this drug because of its side effect profile (more on that in a moment), metoclopramide is the only FDA-approved medication for GP. It works through several mechanisms of action, including inhibiting dopamine-2 (D2) receptors, stimulating 5-HT4 receptors, and promoting release of acetylcholine in the foregut.[71] The net effect is to enhance antral contractions and decrease postprandial fundus relaxation. It does not work beyond the proximal gut, however, and does not help dysmotility in the small bowel or colon (although we still see many people using metoclopramide for ileus where its effects are negligible). In addition to promoting motility, metoclopramide also has direct antiemetic effects by inhibiting D2 and 5-HT3 receptors in the chemoreceptor trigger zone of the medulla oblongata.[71] So, this drug is notable for having both promotility and antiemetic dual effects, which is why metoclopramide remains a popular option for GP

> Metoclopramide has both antiemetic and promotility effects

despite its side effect profile. Most people start with 5-10mg TID before meals and see how it goes from there. If you do prescribe metoclopramide, then it's important to know that the FDA placed a Black Box warning on the drug back in 2009 due to risk of tardive dyskinesia (TD), a side effect characterized by uncontrolled muscle movements in the face, neck, and limbs. The FDA warning restricts use for up to 12 weeks and only in patients under 65 years of age. The highest risk groups for TD include elderly women, diabetics, patients with liver or kidney failure, and patients with concomitant antipsychotic drug therapy. That said, the risk of TD is probably much lower than previously thought.[72] The most comprehensive study to date found a TD risk of around 0.1% per 1,000 patient years, well below the previously estimated 10%-15% per 1,000 patient years.[73] Given the low overall risk of TD coupled with the reality that GP does not just conveniently disappear after 12 weeks of FDA-recommended treatment, some docs extend metoclopramide dosing for more than 3 months. If you plan to use metoclopramide for longer periods, then be sure to confirm that (a) it's really helping (obviously), (b) it is well tolerated, (c) the patient is well-educated about the risks of TD and those discussions are documented in the chart, and (d) you follow the patient carefully and always ask about any adverse reactions. Deciding whether to continue metoclopramide beyond 12 weeks is a decision that should be made carefully and in close communication between doctor and patient.

Domperidone: This is a good alternative to metoclopramide if you can get it. It's not widely available in the US but can be obtained through a special program administered by the FDA. Domperidone outperforms placebo in many forms of GP, including idiopathic, diabetic, and postsurgical GP. Like metoclopramide, domperidone works as a D2 receptor antagonist and has both antiemetic and promotility effects, making it another dual-action

drug for a range of GP symptoms. But unlike metoclopramide, domperidone has minimal penetration
through the blood-brain barrier and is not associated with troubling neurological side effects like TD, making it a
good option to metoclopramide.[74]

Motilin Agonists: The motilin agonists, including erythromycin,
clarithromycin, and azithromycin, promote gastric motility and
can be used for up to 4 weeks in the management of GP. They do
not have an antiemetic effect so these agents are not ideal for managing nausea and vomiting, but they may have short-
term benefits for dysmotility-related symptoms like
postprandial fullness and early satiety. The main
issue with motilin agonists is that patients develop tachyphylaxis after more than a month of use.[75]
Unfortunately, these meds lose their effect and are
therefore not an ideal long-term treatment for GP. They are generally safe, however, as motilin agonists do not cause TD and are not
associated with arrhythmias or cardiovascular mortality.[76]

Prucalopride: This is a highly selective 5-HT4 receptor agonist
that is FDA-cleared for management of chronic constipation. Prucalopride also has effects in the foregut and limited data suggest
evidence of clinical benefit for GP, although the results are not
yet consistent among studies.[77,78] It can help with motility-related
symptoms but has no antiemetic properties, so don't expect it to
help much with nausea and vomiting. For a patient like the woman
described in this vignette, it is reasonable to consider prucalopride
because it can treat both foregut and hindgut symptoms, including
comorbid constipation and bloating.

There are a few other meds that people consider
for GP, but we won't go over those in detail here.
Check out the guidelines for more. But you should
know that central neuromodulators, like tricyclic
antidepressants, have not shown much benefit for

GP and are *not recommended* by the ACG guidelines. Same applies to ghrelin agonists and haloperidol: both are not recommended by the guidelines.

Now, in some instances both dietary and medical therapy are inadequate to relieve symptoms. In those cases, the ACG guidelines suggest considering non-pharmacological treatments, of which there are several listed in **Figure 1.12**. We're going to breeze through these quickly because they are specialized interventions. Check out the guidelines for more detailed information. Here's the lowdown:

Gastric Electrical Stimulation: Also called the gastric "pacemaker," this device may be considered for control of GP symptoms as a humanitarian use device by the FDA. It is reserved for patients with medically refractory symptoms and the existing data remain mixed in terms of clinical benefit.

Botulinum Injection: For years, endoscopists have been experimenting with injecting botulinum toxin into the pylorus for people with GP. The goal is to limit outflow resistance by paralyzing the pylorus, hopefully leading to reduced GP symptoms. Unfortunately, randomized trials have not borne this out and the ACG guidelines do not currently recommend this therapy for patients with GP.

Intrapyloric botulinum injection is not recommended

Gastric Per-Oral Endoscopic Myotomy (G-POEM): G-POEM is reserved for the toughest cases where dietary and medical therapy have largely failed. Here, the endoscopist performs a per-oral pyloric myotomy to reduce gastric outflow obstruction. When it works, it works great. But it doesn't work in everyone. The guidelines indicate that using the EndoFLIP (endoluminal functional lumen imaging probe) device may be useful to select patients for G-POEM. EndoFLIP allows endoscopic measurement of pyloric diameter, distensibility, and compliance. When these figures are out of whack, then it can help justify G-POEM and appears to guide

Consider EndoFLIP to guide use of G-POEM

appropriate use of the procedure. Further technical details can be found in the guidelines, but for now, just know that the ACG recommends EndoFLIP evaluation to characterize pyloric function and predict outcomes after peroral pyloromyotomy.

Case 1.9: Management of Constipation

A 68-year-old man presents for evaluation in your clinic, which is his first medical appointment in several years. He mentions that he has had more than 20 years of constipation associated with lower abdominal bloating. He typically has about 2 to 3 bowel movements per week, which relieve his bloating sensation. However, he feels that his symptoms have slowly progressed over the past several months with decreased stool frequency and increased bloating. He has been on a "high fiber diet" and drinks plenty of liquids. There has been no abdominal pain, weight loss, hematochezia, appetite problems or fatigue. He feels well otherwise and still partakes in spin cycling for one hour every other day. His physical examination is unremarkable. A complete blood count and laboratory investigations are also normal. He previously received a colonoscopy 4 years ago that was unremarkable and has no independent risk factors for colon cancer. He would like to know what can be done to help.

Know your guidelines!

1. What is the next diagnostic step?
2. What therapeutic options should be considered?

Case 1.9: What do the guidelines say?

Source: Joint ACG/AGA 2023 Pharmacological Management of Chronic Idiopathic Constipation Guidelines

We thought about starting this chapter with a constipation pun, but it just didn't come out right. This was too hard to pass up

Okay, onto the ACG constipation guidelines, which are a joint document written in partnership with the AGA.[79] To be clear, the guidelines do not address the diagnostic workup for constipation, so we'll only mention testing briefly. Just as with the IBS-C and anorectal disorder guidelines, anyone old enough for colon cancer screening should get a colonoscopy (or other form of colon cancer screening) if they need it, regardless of whether they have constipation. Of course, if a patient has alarm features along with constipation, such as unintended weight loss, rectal bleeding, or iron deficiency anemia, then they should receive a colonoscopy (and likely an upper endoscopy, too) regardless of age. The patient in the vignette has no alarm features and had a normal colonoscopy 4 years ago, so a repeat colonoscopy is not recommended at this time; he's not due for another 6 years, as we'll discuss in the chapter on GI cancer screening guidelines.

But the ACG/AGA guidelines are all about treatment. So, let's figure out how to manage this patient.

Fiber Supplementation: The guidelines recommend that patients with chronic idiopathic constipation (CIC) be initially considered for fiber supplementation, although the authors readily admit the evidence is far from overwhelming. You'll recall that fiber is categorized as either soluble or insoluble based on its ability to form a gel-like substance in water (we also covered this in the IBS-C discussion earlier in the book). Wheat bran is a classic insoluble fiber, whereas psyllium is considered to be a soluble fiber (although it does Wheat bran is insoluble, oat bran is soluble (got it?) have insoluble components) with some prebiotic effects, too. Oat bran is also soluble (not to be confused with insoluble wheat bran).

These various forms of fiber have different effects on both physiology and clinical outcomes. Soluble fiber traps water and softens poop, whereas insoluble fiber just makes your poop all fat and bulky. Nobody wants to poop all fat and bulky. So, suggesting to a patient that they simply "increase fiber intake" is not exactly helpful. In fact, a review article by McRorie and colleagues suggests that generically recommending fiber for CIC is like recommending someone "increase pill intake without regard to therapeutic or adverse effects."[80] It's sort of a useless instruction.

In this vignette, the patient refers to consuming a "high fiber diet," but it will be important to understand *which* fiber products he is consuming and *how much* is being consumed. This is important because the data are pretty clear (that's right: data *are*, not data *is*) that soluble fiber—namely psyllium—can be reasonably effective for CIC, whereas insoluble fiber is generally less effective or, in some studies, not effective at all. In fact, wheat bran can actually decrease stool water content and *harden*—not soften—stool when consumed as a finely-ground powder, whereas it may have some benefits when consumed as a coarse product. It is also generally recommended to consume around 20-30g of fiber per day, as tolerated, to optimize its physiologic effects. However, fiber can also cause flatulence which limits its acceptability and undermines adherence. The guidelines do recommend "adequate hydration" when consuming fiber to help avoid stool hardening, but acknowledge this advice is not very evidence based. After all, we don't poop out water, we pee it out. So, increasing water intake will mainly lead to more pee, not more poo (that's right, we keep saying "pee" and "poo" in a peer-reviewed book; you'll just have to roll with it).

Polyethylene glycol (PEG) products: You will recall from earlier in the chapter that PEG is not great for treating IBS-C. We promised we'd come back to PEG and CIC, so, here we are. Let's talk PEG.

Our formal scientific assessment is that PEG is pretty bad ass. It's easy to administer, has no nasty taste (or *any* taste, for that matter), is highly effective, available over the counter, can be flexibly dosed, and is well tolerated with few significant adverse effects. PEG is approved at a dose of 17 g daily, which comes as a capful of white powder mixed into whatever beverage the patient prefers. Data indicate that PEG not only improves spontaneous bowel movement (SBM) frequency, but can also produce the nirvana-like *complete* spontaneous bowel movements (CSBMs) in which patients not only pass their stool, but it comes out completely, without a sense of partial evacuation, leading to a highly satisfying poop (there, we said the p-word again).[81] Studies show that PEG is durably effective over 6 months of use and is similarly effective as secretagogues like tegaserod and prucalopride.[82,83] Finally, there is no difference in side effects between PEG and placebo, which is a rarity among effective medicines (although it can still cause abdominal distension, loose stools, flatulence, and nausea if overused). Bottom line: we're PEG fans and would consider it for this patient.

Magnesium Oxide (MgO): Like all osmotic laxatives, MgO creates an osmotic gradient and passively pulls fluid into the lumen to soften stool. The guideline authors indicate that they have "very low certainty" that MgO does much, which is not exactly a ringing endorsement. Also, be very careful using MgO in patients with renal insufficiency, particularly when the creatinine clearance falls below 20mg/dL. On the other hand, MgO is a lot cheaper than PEG (which, by the way, seems way too expensive for a simple plastic powder, but we digress), indicating that it still has a role for some people, particularity those with limited access to pharmacotherapies.

Lactulose: The guidelines are sort of, well, "*meh...*" about lactulose, a synthetic disaccharide that also works as an osmotic laxative. This syrupy substance is FDA approved for constipation at a dose of 10-20g per day, although the existing trials are small and limited. The guidelines indicate "very low certainty" that lactulose is effective, but make the bold statement that "use of lactulose" is suggested "over management without lactulose." We interpret that to mean that it's reasonable to prescribe lactulose if you're on a desert island with no other constipation meds at your disposal. The most common complications of lactulose are bloating and flatulence, as one would expect when ingesting a sugar.

Bisacodyl: This agent appears to work directly on the colonic mucosa to kick-start high amplitude propagating contractions. As a stimulant laxative, bisacodyl can get things moving quickly and is often used as "rescue therapy" for patients who need a helping hand. Because bisacodyl can really crank the colon, it's understandable that abdominal pain, cramping, and diarrhea are the most common adverse consequences of treatment. For this reason, the guidelines recommend prescribing 5mg orally rather than the 10mg dose used in published trials. Because side effects are so common, it is generally not advised to use bisacodyl as a long-term agent, in contrast to its use as a rescue agent when primary therapies need temporary augmentation.

Senna: Senna is another stimulant laxative, but unlike bisacodyl, the guidelines conclude that it's "probably appropriate" to use senna longer term if needed. It's a low cost, easily available treatment with reasonable data for effectiveness, making senna an appealing first-line pharmacotherapy for managing chronic idiopathic constipation (CIC). As with bisacodyl, senna is associated with abdominal pain and cramping, particularly when using higher doses.

Lubiprostone: We covered this agent in the IBS-C chapter earlier in the book, but will provide a quick summary here. Lubiprostone is a unique agent that increases intestinal chloride secretion by activating type 2 chloride channels. Approved by the FDA for management of CIC, this prostaglandin E1 analogue improves stool frequency and form although it's associated with nausea in a dose-dependent fashion and may cause excessive diarrhea. Despite that, it's a well-tolerated medication overall with discontinuation rates of only 5% in clinical trials.

Linaclotide: We also covered this drug earlier in the book, but as a quick refresher, this is a guanylate cyclase-C agonist that triggers water secretion into the colon and enhances motility. Importantly, linaclotide also reduces symptoms of bloating, discomfort and pain in IBS-C trials while improving CIC symptoms. It's important to know the dosing is different for CIC than for IBS-C, with approved dosing of either 72mg or 145mg daily for the former condition, but 290 mg for the latter. The most common side effect is diarrhea, although severe diarrhea leading to discontinuation is rare, occurring in just under 5% of clinical trial participants.

> Remember the dose of linaclotide is different for CIC than IBS-C

Plecanatide: This is another guanylate cyclase-C agonist approved by the FDA for management of CIC. The usual dose is 3mg daily. As with linaclotide, diarrhea is the most common side effect.

> Plecanatide headache usually resolves after a few days

Prucalopride: Not to be confused with plecanatide, prucalopride is a highly selective agonist of serotonin 5-HT4 receptors in the colon. The starting dose is 2mg daily. This is a highly effective medication that improves GI symptoms and quality of life among patients with CIC, although it is limited by side effects like headache, abdominal pain, nausea, and diarrhea. These symptoms usually arise upon starting therapy and tend to resolve within a few days, so patients should be aware of this predictable sequence before prematurely discontinuing therapy.

Okay, and with that, we end our review of the ACG neurogastroenterology and motility guidelines. Onto the esophagus—after you answer some questions on the next few pages, which we expect you to get 100% correct!

Neurogastroenterology and Motility Guidelines Quiz

1. How frequently must patients experience abdominal pain to meet Rome IV criteria for IBS?

    a) $\geq$1 day per month
    b) $\geq$1 day per week
    c) $\geq$3 days per week
    d) Daily

2. What is the recommended dose of glucose for use in a glucose breath test?

    a) 25g
    b) 50g
    c) 75g
    d) 100g

3. Which of the following breath hydrogen thresholds defines SIBO based on breath testing?

    a) $\geq$10ppm rise by 60 min
    b) $\geq$10ppm rise by 90 min
    c) $\geq$20ppm rise by 60 min
    d) $\geq$20ppm rise by 90 min

4. Presence of which of the following intestinal gasses is associated with diarrhea?

    a) Hydrogen
    b) Hydrogen sulfide
    c) Methane
    d) Carbon dioxide

5. Each the following is required to meet Rome IV criteria for IBS EXCEPT:

    a) Abdominal pain
    b) Change in stool frequency or form
    c) Abdominal discomfort

6. What is the recommended dose of lactulose for use in a lactu-
    lose breath test?

    a) 5g
    b) 10g
    c) 15g
    d) 20g

7. Which of the following breath methane thresholds defines
    IMO based on breath testing?

    a) $\geq$10ppm rise at any time
    b) $\geq$10ppm rise by 30 min
    c) $\geq$10ppm rise by 60 min
    d) $\geq$10ppm rise by 90 min

8. Which of the following is true about the treatment of SIBO
    and IMO?

    a) FMT is recommended for *M. smithii* overgrowth
    b) Probiotics are recommended for SIBO
    c) There is no role for a low FODMAP diet for SIBO
    d) Rifaximin and neomycin is an effective combo therapy for
        IMO

9. Which of the following thresholds defines SIBO based on cul-
    ture of duodenal aspirate?

    a) $\geq$10^2 CFU/mL
    b) $\geq$10^3 CFU/mL
    c) $\geq$10^4 CFU/mL
    d) $\geq$10^5 CFU/mL

10. Which of the following is true about breath testing?

    a) Most ingested glucose passes into the colon
    b) Glucose is less specific than lactulose for SIBO
    c) Lactulose is a rapidly absorbed sugar

d) Lactulose breath test can be falsely positive if there is rapid intestinal transit

11. Which of the following is the most common type of methanogen found in IMO?

    a) *S. bovus*
    b) *Lactobacillus*
    c) *M. smithii*
    d) *E. coli*

12. The ACG guidelines recommend all the following tests for IBS EXCEPT?

    a) ESR
    b) CRP
    c) Fecal calprotectin
    d) Fecal lactoferrin

13. All the following are true about testing for celiac disease in IBS EXCEPT?

    a) Testing is not indicated for patients with IBS-C
    b) Testing for quantitative IgA level can help reduce the risk of false negative anti-TTG IgA
    c) IBS patients are 4.5x more likely than controls to have positive celiac serologies
    d) It is cost-effective to routinely test for celiac disease in IBS

14. Which of the following is true about performing colonoscopy in patients with IBS?

    a) A negative colonoscopy tends to reassure patients with IBS and improve their quality of life
    b) Colonoscopy with biopsy should be recommended early in patients with IBS-D to rule-out microscopic colitis
    c) The risk of finding colon cancer in patients with IBS is roughly 0.1%
    d) Colonoscopy is the guideline-preferred test to distinguish IBD from IBS

15. All the following are risk factors for post-infectious IBS EX-
CEPT:

    a) Female sex
    b) Older age
    c) History of anxiety
    d) Longer duration of index infection

16. The risk of developing post-infectious IBS after an intestinal
bacterial infection is:

    a) 3%
    b) 7%
    c) 11%
    d) 15%

17. An "IBS" patient has intermittent pain attacks, hyponatremia,
neuropathic and neuropsychiatric symptoms, and elevated
transaminases. Which of the following conditions are you most
worried about?

    a) Carcinoid syndrome
    b) Acute intermittent porphyria
    c) VIPoma
    d) Hereditary angioedema

18. All the following are examples of FODMAPs EXCEPT?

    a) Fructans
    b) Gluten
    c) Fructose
    d) Polyols
    e) Galacto-oligosaccharides

19. Beans are a common source of which type of FODMAP?

    a) Fructans
    b) Fructose
    c) Polyols
    d) Galacto-oligosaccharides

e) Lactose

20. Garlic and onions are common sources of which type of FOD-
MAP?

    a) Fructans
    b) Fructose
    c) Polyols
    d) Galacto-oligosaccharides
    e) Lactose

21. Peaches and cherries are common sources of which type of
FODMAP?

    a) Fructans
    b) Fructose
    c) Polyols
    d) Galacto-oligosaccharides
    e) Lactose

22. What is the minimum time to trial a low FODMAP diet before
determining if it is clinically effective?

    a) 1 week
    b) 2 weeks
    c) 4 weeks
    d) 8 weeks

23. Which of the following is an example of an insoluble fiber that
is not effective for managing IBS?

    a) Oat bran
    b) Wheat bran
    c) Psyllium
    d) Barley

24. The recommended daily dose of soluble fiber for IBS is:

    a) 10g per day
    b) 15g per day
    c) 20g per day
    d) 25g per day

25. Which of the following medications is recommended by the ACG IBS guidelines?

    a) Dicyclomine
    b) Colesevelam
    c) Loperamide
    d) Eluxadoline

26. All the following treatments are recommended by the ACG IBS guidelines EXCEPT:

    a) Linaclotide
    b) Peppermint oil
    c) Probiotics
    d) Lubiprostone

27. Which of the following TCAs has the most prominent anticholinergic side effects?

    a) Imipramine
    b) Amitriptyline
    c) Desipramine
    d) Nortriptyline

28. Alosetron works on which of the following forms of serotonin?

    a) 5-HT1
    b) 5-HT2
    c) 5-HT3
    d) 5-HT4

29. Lubiprostone is:

    a) A GC-C agonist
    b) A chloride channel agonist
    c) A mixed opioid receptor agonist/antagonist
    d) A smooth muscle relaxant

30. Which of the following is a known adverse effect of eluxadoline?

a) Pancreatitis
b) Diarrhea
c) Hepatitis
d) Ischemic colitis

31. What percentage of IBS-D patients have evidence of bile acid malabsorption on Se-HCAT testing?

a) 8%
b) 18%
c) 28%
d) 38%

32. What is the minimum time one must have epigastric pain to meet ACG criteria for "dyspepsia"?

a) 1 month
b) 2 months
c) 3 months
d) 4 months

33. At what age is endoscopy warranted in the diagnostic evaluation of dyspepsia?

a) $\geq$50 years
b) $\geq$55 years
c) $\geq$60 years
d) $\geq$65 years

34. According to the ACG guideline algorithm, when should an endoscopy be performed for a patient <60 years old who has dyspepsia and concurrent GI alarm features?

a) At the time of diagnosis
b) If $\geq$50 years old
c) If $\geq$55 years old
d) Endoscopy should not be performed

35. What is the first treatment step for a patient with functional dyspepsia?

    a) Administer a PPI trial
    b) Administer a prokinetic
    c) Test for *H. pylori* and treat if positive
    d) Administer a TCA

36. Which of the following symptoms reliably distinguishes between a defecatory disorder and slow-transit constipation?

    a) Need for manual maneuvers
    b) Sense of incomplete evacuation
    c) Sense of anorectal blockage
    d) No symptoms reliably distinguish between entities

37. Which of the following is the most appropriate next step for a patient with symptoms suggestive of a defecatory disorder?

    a) Advise to use a footstool during defecation
    b) Balloon expulsion test
    c) Anorectal manometry
    d) Barium defecography

38. What is the recommended balloon volume for use in a balloon expulsion test?

    a) 30cc
    b) 50cc
    c) 70cc
    d) 90cc

39. What is the minimum number of anorectal biofeedback sessions needed before determining clinical efficacy for a patient with dyssynergic defecation?

    a) 2 sessions
    b) 4 sessions
    c) 8 sessions
    d) 10 sessions

40. A patient with symptoms suggestive of a defecatory disorder fails conservative management. What is the most appropriate next step?

   a) Balloon expulsion test
   b) Anorectal manometry
   c) Combined balloon expulsion test and anorectal manometry
   d) Defecography
   e) Colonic radio-opaque marker study

41. The overall age-adjusted prevalence of fecal incontinence in the United States is:

   a) 1%
   b) 5%
   c) 9%
   d) 13%

42. Which of the following is a common mechanism of passive incontinence?

   a) External anal sphincter tear
   b) Pudendal nerve damage
   c) Autonomic neuropathy
   d) Ulcerative proctitis

43. Which of the following is the most appropriate initial step for suspected levator ani syndrome?

   a) Perform anorectal manometry
   b) Begin treatment with topical calcium channel blocker
   c) Intersphincteric botulinum toxin injection
   d) Begin treatment with topical nitroglycerin
   e) High dose NSAIDs

44. Which of the following is true about the internal anal sphincter?

   a) It is comprised of smooth muscle
   b) It governs squeeze pressure
   c) It is innervated by the pudendal nerve
   d) It is anatomically lateral to the external anal sphincter

45. You perform a perianal pinprick test in a patient with fecal incontinence. The anal wink is not elicited. Which of the following is the most appropriate next step?

   a) Perform anorectal manometry
   b) Refer for needle EMG testing of the anal sphincter
   c) Begin anorectal biofeedback training
   d) Order MRI of the lumbosacral spine

46. All the following are appropriate for initial management of mild fecal incontinence symptoms EXCEPT:

   a) Loperamide
   b) Anorectal manometry
   c) Pelvic floor exercises
   d) Education about the causes of incontinence

47. A woman with fecal incontinence fails conservative therapy. Anorectal manometry and EUS reveal a weak external anal sphincter but no disruption to the muscular ring. What treatment is most appropriate?

   a) Anal plug
   b) Perianal injection of bulking agent
   c) Anorectal biofeedback therapy
   d) Intravaginal balloon
   e) Sacral nerve stimulation

48. What percentage of patients with gastroparesis (GP) in referral centers report abdominal pain?

   a) 10%
   b) 30%
   c) 50%
   d) 70%
   e) 90%

49. Which of the following is the most common cause of GP?

   a) Diabetes
   b) Medications
   c) Postsurgical
   d) Idiopathic
   e) Neurodegenerative disorders

50. Which of the following classes of medications can delay gastric emptying?

   a) GLP-1 agonists
   b) Motilin receptor agonists
   c) Cholinergics
   d) Dopamine-2 receptor antagonists
   e) 5-HT4 agonists

51. A 35-year-old patient had recurrent postprandial fullness, nausea, vomiting, and abdominal pain. Which of the following is the next step in managing this patient?

   a) Initiate a small particle, low fat diet
   b) Conduct a 4-hour solid phase gastric emptying study
   c) Begin metoclopramide
   d) Begin a tricyclic antidepressant
   e) Perform upper endoscopy

52. Which of the following is true about scintigraphic gastric emptying for diagnosing GP?

   a) A 90-minute solid phase exam is adequate
   b) The test requires patients to consume a high fat, radiolabeled eggbeater meal
   c) Scans should be obtained every 10 minutes during the course of the study
   d) The test is considered positive if there is $\leq 90\%$ emptying after 4 hours
   e) It is acceptable for patients using cannabinoids to continue while preparing for the test

53. Which of the following is an independent risk factor for developing tardive dyskinesia from metoclopramide?

    a) Age under 65 years
    b) Male gender
    c) Diabetes
    d) Hypertension
    e) Exceeding 8 weeks of therapy

54. Which of the following most closely reflects the true rate of tardive dyskinesia per 1,000 patient years of metoclopramide use?

    a) 0.1%
    b) 1%
    c) 5%
    d) 10%
    e) 15%

55. Which of the following is true about medical therapies for GP?

    a) Metoclopramide works as a dopamine-2 receptor agonist
    b) Domperidone rapidly crosses the blood-brain barrier and increases risk of tardive dyskinesia
    c) Prucalopride is a highly selective 5-HT3 receptor agonist
    d) Motilin agonists should only be used for short term relief of GP due to risk of tachyphylaxis

56. Bisacodyl works by:

    a) Activating type 2 chloride channels
    b) Activating 5-HT4 receptors in the colon
    c) Mimicking the effects of prostaglandin E1
    d) Triggering high-amplitude prorogating contractions in the colon
    e) Agonizing GCC receptors

57. Lactulose works by:

    a) Activating type 2 chloride channels
    b) Activating 5-HT4 receptors in the colon
    c) Mimicking the effects of prostaglandin E1

d) Triggering high-amplitude prorogating contractions in the colon

e) Passively drawing fluid into the colonic lumen

58. Plecanatide works by:

a) Activating type 2 chloride channels

b) Activating 5-HT4 receptors in the colon

c) Agonizing GC-C receptors

d) Triggering high-amplitude prorogating contractions in the colon

e) Passively drawing fluid into the colonic lumen

59. Which of the following is true about prucalopride?

a) It is GC-C receptor agonist

b) It is FDA approved for management of IBS-C and CIC

c) Headache is a common early side effect that tends to wane after several days of use

d) Nausea occurs as a consequence of prostaglandin effects

60. Which of the following is true about *Guide to the Guidelines Volume I*:

a) Reading this book might cause some people to feel gassy, dispirited, or both

b) This book would be more fun to read if written in pig Latin

c) It is unusual for a peer-reviewed book to use the word "poop" 8 times in a chapter

d) Not all of the jokes in this book are as funny as the authors might think

e) All of the above are true

Answers to Neurogastroenterology and Motility Guidelines Quiz

1.	B	21.	C	41.	C
2.	C	22.	B	42.	C
3.	D	23.	B	43.	A
4.	B	24.	D	44.	A
5.	C	25.	D	45.	D
6.	B	26.	C	46.	B
7.	A	27.	B	47.	C
8.	D	28.	C	48.	E
9.	B	29.	B	49.	D
10.	D	30.	A	50.	A
11.	C	31.	C	51.	E
12.	A	32.	A	52.	D
13.	A	33.	C	53.	C
14.	C	34.	D	54.	A
15.	B	35.	C	55.	D
16.	C	36.	D	56.	D
17.	B	37.	A	57.	E
18.	B	38.	B	58.	B
19.	D	39.	B	59.	C
20.	A	40.	C	60.	E

Chapter Two

Down The Hatch

Esophagus Guidelines

Got GERD? Lots of people do. Either you have GERD, or you know someone else who does. Or both. So, let's begin our journey through the ACG esophageal guidelines with a discussion about this common and burdensome condition. And here's the deal: every GI doc knows about GERD, but when pressed, many of us realize that our knowledge is outdated. It's like whatever we learned as a trainee lingers within us while the science of GERD continues to evolve. We'll clean that up in this chapter.

While we're talking about the esophagus, it is also important to stay on top of the latest guidelines about esophageal motility disorders. Be honest. How well do you know the Chicago Classification for achalasia? Do high resolution manometry tracings make you nuts? Do they look more like Rorschach tests than, well, whatever they're supposed to look like? In this chapter, we'll introduce some easy ways to learn esophageal motility tracings. Stay tuned.

In the meantime, let's get started by going down the hatch and exploring the latest on GERD.

Case 2.1: Management of Uninvestigated GERD

A 63-year-old man has been experiencing heartburn after eating spicy foods. Due to the indigestion, he has maintained a bland diet at home and has avoided eating out. There has been no dysphagia, odynophagia, early satiety, vomiting, abdominal pain, weight loss or melena. He has taken over-the-counter acid reducers (calcium carbonate) without complete relief. Physical examination is unremarkable. His laboratory tests including a complete blood count are normal.

Know your guidelines!

What should be done next?

Case 2.1: What do the guidelines say?

Source: ACG 2021 GERD Guidelines

"A lot has changed, much remains the same."

That's the first line of the ACG GERD guidelines. Although GERD is a well-understood condition with widely used and effective therapies, the science of GERD continues to evolve; it is important to keep up with the latest research. Here, and in the next few vignettes, we will summarize the most current ACG guidance on GERD management.

Okay, so what is GERD? The ACG offers this definition:[84]

> *GERD is the condition in which reflux of gastric contents into the esophagus results in symptoms and/or complications. GERD is objectively defined by the presence of characteristic mucosal injury seen at endoscopy and/or abnormal esophageal acid exposure demonstrated on a reflux monitoring study.*

This definition means that gastroesophageal reflux (GER) is different from **GERD**. Acid might reflux into the esophagus, but unless and until it causes trouble, GER is not GERD. The "D" in GERD implies there is disease, or "lack of ease," so to speak. That means reflux is causing symptoms, like heartburn, regurgitation, or chest pain, or is leading to complications like erosive esophagitis, peptic strictures, or Barrett's esophagus (more on Barrett's later).

Although the causes of GERD are not enumerated in the ACG guidelines, we thought it might be useful to review the top-to-bottom process we follow in clinic when evaluating a patient with GERD symptoms. Follow along with **Figure 2.1**.

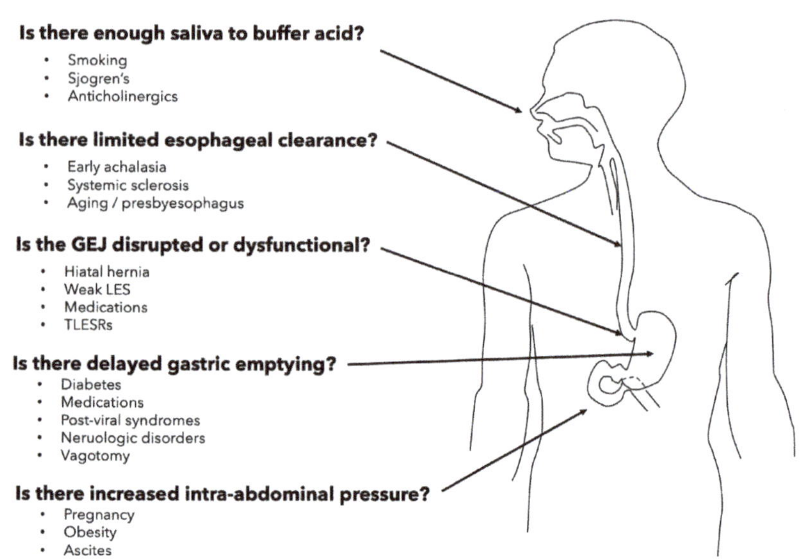

Figure 2.1: Mechanisms of increased esophageal acid exposure. For each patient you see with GERD symptoms, consider following this top-to-bottom mental routine to consider underlying mechanisms that may be causing acid reflux.

We start by thinking about the mouth, then progress down the esophagus, then consider the lower esophageal sphincter (LES) and gastroesophageal junction (GEJ), then the stomach, and finally consider any contributing factors *around* the stomach. If you follow this routine every time, then it will help you think broadly about GERD rather than, say, reflexively jumping to a PPI discussion without considering why your patient might have GERD symptoms.

Starting with the mouth, ask yourself if there is any reason the patient might not be producing enough saliva to buffer esophageal acid. Are they taking an anticholinergic? Or have signs of Sjogren's? Is the patient a long-term smoker? Remember that smoking can diminish saliva production.

Remember that early achalasia and EoE can both mimic GERD

Next comes the esophagus. Could there be defective esophageal clearance? Are there early signs of achalasia? Or systemic sclerosis? Has aging led to slow esophageal peristalsis? Might there be underlying eosinophilic esophagitis (EoE) mimicking GERD?

Next comes the gastroesophageal junction (GEJ). Could there be a hiatal hernia? Might the lower esophageal sphincter (LES) be weak? Is the patient taking any medications or substances that relax the LES, like calcium channel blockers, progesterone, anticholinergics, or peppermint oil? Could there be transient LES relaxations (TLESRs) leading to frequent acid exposure? Fun fact: TLESRs are the most common mechanism of GERD.

Then shift your attention to the stomach. Is it emptying correctly? Could there be gastroparesis from diabetes, anticholinergic medications, post-viral syndromes, neurological disorders, vagotomy, or a paraneoplastic process, like can be seen with small cell lung cancer? Might there be excessive acid production, either from a common condition like antrum-predominant *H. pylori* infection, or a rare condition like Zollinger-Ellison syndrome?

What about extrinsic conditions *around* the stomach? Is anything increasing intra-abdominal pressure? Is there ascites? Obesity? Is the patient pregnant?

We find this top-to-bottom routine to be extremely useful. It allows us to stay focused on seeking mechanisms in lieu of simply prescribing a PPI or going straight to endoscopy without thinking critically. You might still prescribe a PPI or do an endoscopy, but at least you will devote thought to ruling out potentially modifiable risk factors or other underlying conditions.

So, what do the guidelines say to do next for this vignette? Are any diagnostic tests needed at this stage? Or is it okay to jump straight to therapy? The answer depends on whether there are alarm features, including dysphagia, unintended weight loss, GI bleeding, vomiting, or iron deficiency anemia. If any alarm features are present, then upper endoscopy is warranted, regardless of age. The patient in this vignette does not have alarm features, so endoscopy is not (yet) warranted.

Also *be careful not to miss underlying coronary artery disease*. For patients who present with chest pain, with or without other classic GERD symptoms, it is vital to rule out heart disease. Be sure to refer patients to a cardiologist if you're worried.

If there are no alarm features or concerns about heart disease, and assuming the symptoms are severe enough to negatively affect quality of life, then further evaluation is warranted. But you do not need to perform an upper endoscopy at this stage. Instead, you should follow the algorithm shown in **Figure 2.2**. [84]

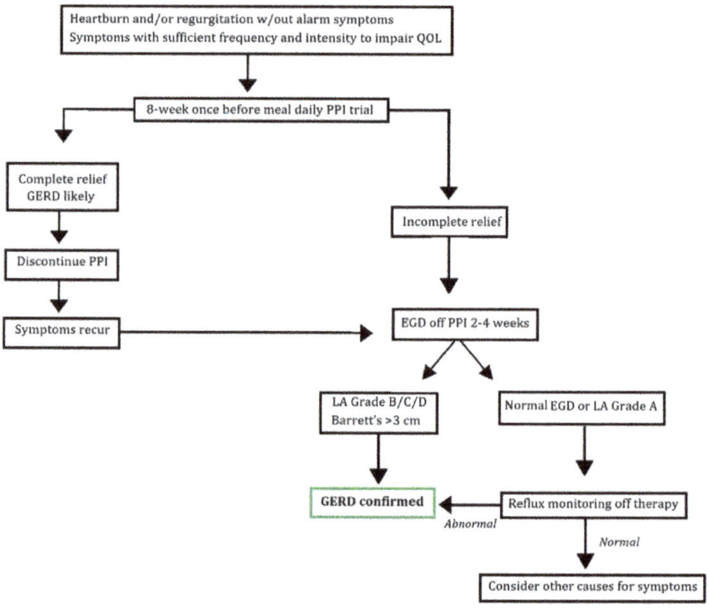

Figure 2.2: ACG Diagnostic Algorithm for GERD symptoms without alarm features.[84]

First, start with an 8-week trial of once-daily therapy with a proton pump inhibitor (PPI) before the first meal of the day. Notice that it says *once per day*. For some reason, we see nuclear doses of PPIs prescribed all the time, like 40mg BID for regular old GERD. That's Zollinger Ellison dosing! There is no need to jump straight to high dose PPIs at this stage and the guidelines make a point of highlighting the risks of long-term, high-dose PPI therapy (more on that later).

The idea behind an 8-week PPI trial is that it's a diagnostic test, unto itself, not just a therapeutic trial. If GERD symptoms improve after a trial of PPIs, then it suggests the underlying condition is indeed GERD. However, there are limitations to this approach. The PPI test is only 78% sensitive and 54% specific for GERD compared to the gold standard of using endoscopy and pH monitoring.[85] So, although using a diagnostic PPI test is pragmatic and cost-effective compared to more invasive testing, it's not perfect.

If the patient feels better after the PPI trial, then it suggests underlying GERD and the trial can be discontinued. If the symptoms recur, which is often the case, then the guidelines support use of upper endoscopy. Similarly, if the PPI trial doesn't work at all, then endoscopy is also warranted.

Here's a key point: before performing diagnostic upper endoscopy for GERD symptoms, it is ideal to first discontinue PPIs for 2-4 weeks. This maneuver will increase the yield of endoscopy by revealing erosive esophagitis, a diagnostic biomarker of GERD that might otherwise be suppressed by PPIs. In addition, PPIs can sometimes obscure Barrett's esophagus by causing squamous mucosa overgrowth. They might also cover up evidence of EoE. You don't want to miss these conditions because of a false negative study. If the patient needs treatment during this PPI-free period, then the guidelines recommend using antacids.

What should you look for during an upper endoscopy for GERD? Lots of things. First, look for evidence of erosive esophagitis and, if present, use the Los Angeles classification system to grade the injury (see **Figure 2.3**). If you can't memorize this system, then put it on the wall of your endoscopy suite and use it liberally.

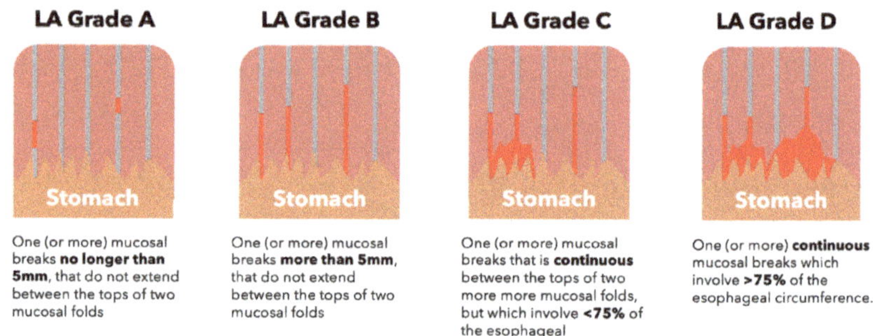

Figure 2.3: Los Angeles Classification System for Erosive Esophagitis. Designed by B. Spiegel.

Next, look for a hiatal hernia. If you see one, then describe it carefully, ideally using a standardized score like the Hill grading system shown in **Figure 2.4**. You might throw this up on your endoscopy suite wall, too, if it helps.

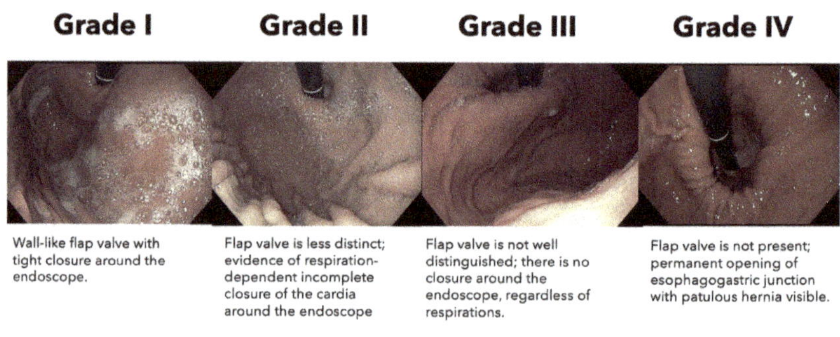

Figure 2.4: Hill Grading System for Hiatal Hernias. Image source: Kavya Reddy, MD.

Also look for salmon-colored mucosa suggestive of Barrett's esophagus. If you see it, then describe the abnormal segment using the circumference and maximum length ("C&M") system, which we will cover in more detail in a later vignette.

While you're in there, look for any signs of EoE, like rings or furrows. Check for signs of altered motility, such as excessive tortuosity of the esophageal body. Get a sense if there might be early achalasia, evidenced by a dilated esophagus or difficulty passing through the GEJ. See if there are signs of gastroparesis, including retained gastric contents. Look for Zollinger-Ellison clues, like thick gastric folds, excessive gastric juice, or multiple ulcers (especially post-bulbar ulcers). In short, *think broadly*: don't just scope-in and scope-out!

After the endoscopy: Okay, so either the endoscopy will show clear cut evidence of GERD, or it won't. By "clear cut evidence," the guidelines mean that you either found LA *Class <u>B</u> or greater* erosive esophagitis, and/or you discovered a segment of Barrett's esophagus that *exceeds 3cm in length*. But if you encountered a normal EGD or only LA Class A esophagitis, then you cannot yet confirm a diagnosis of GERD. In that case, reflux monitoring is indicated.

Key points about reflux monitoring: Reflux monitoring can be a pain to set up and perform (mainly, for the patient), but it enables direct assessment of esophageal acid exposure and is a pathognomonic test for GERD. The 2 methods of reflux monitoring include use of a wireless telemetry capsule attached to the distal esophageal mucosa for 48-96 hours, or use of a transnasal catheter for 24 hours. The wireless capsule is much more comfortable for patients than the transnasal catheter but requires endoscopic placement. In contrast, the transnasal catheter can employ both pH-metry and impedance, meaning it can discriminate among acidic, weakly acidic, and non-acidic refluxate. That capability is helpful to distinguish acid reflux from, say, bile reflux. In contrast, the wireless capsule cannot make that distinction and is limited to measuring acid.

Both types of monitoring will measure the *acid exposure time* (AET), which is the percentage of time when the esophageal pH falls below 4. When AET exceeds 4% of the study duration, then it indicates pathologic acid reflux. Reflux monitoring can also evaluate the relationship between symptom events and reflux events using 2 metrics: *the symptom index* (SI) and the *symptom association probability* (SAP). The SI measures the proportion of reflux episodes that trigger a symptom; if that value exceeds 50%, then the SI is positive. The SAP is a bit more involved and requires calculating a p-value for the concurrence of symptoms and reflux events over the course of the monitoring period. If the SAP exceeds 95%, then it's considered positive. There is no intrinsic advantage of the SI over the SAP, so both can be evaluated side-by-side.

Here's the eternal question about reflux monitoring: *should it be performed on, or off PPIs?* This question comes up a lot. Let's break down the answer here. Check out **Figure 2.2** again. You'll notice that it says to perform reflux monitoring *off* therapy when attempting to establish the diagnosis of GERD. Ideally, PPIs should be *stopped for 7 days* prior to reflux monitoring. And that's that. But is there ever a reason to perform reflux monitoring *on* therapy? Yes, but only in patients who already have an established diagnosis of GERD. In that situation, you might consider reflux monitoring *on* treatment if there are persistent symptoms *despite PPI therapy.* That makes sense because in that scenario you want to determine if the PPIs are truly lowering acid exposure. Also, if you conduct transnasal catheter monitoring with impedance while on PPIs, then you can distinguish acidic vs weakly acidic (or non-acidic) reflux. We'll address issue of poor PPI response in the next vignette.

Case 2.2: Management of Persistent GERD Despite PPIs

A 43-year-old woman presents to your clinic for follow up due to persistent heartburn for the past several years. She smokes one pack of cigarettes daily and has a body mass index of 34. She describes a retrosternal burning sensation which occurs soon after eating. There has been no abdominal pain, dysphagia, nausea, vomiting, early satiety, or weight loss.

She had seen her primary care provider a few months ago for this complaint and had labs drawn, which showed a normal CBC, complete metabolic panel, and ferritin. She was started on omeprazole 40mg daily with modest but not complete resolution of her symptoms.

On initial consult, you advised holding the omeprazole for 4 weeks and performed an EGD with a wireless telemetry capsule attachment. The EGD shows an endoscopically normal esophagus and stomach without a hiatal hernia. The reading from the reflux monitoring reveals that the acid exposure time was 7% of the study duration.

Know your guidelines!

What should you advise next?

Case 2.2: What do the guidelines say?

Source: ACG 2021 GERD Guidelines

We hate to be the bearers of bad news, but PPIs don't always work out as planned ☺. This patient has evidence of pathologic acid reflux on monitoring, but PPIs are not relieving her symptoms. So, we need to discuss why PPIs sometimes fall short and what to do about it.

Before we get there, it's important to first discuss non-pharmacological treatments for GERD. If we rely on meds alone without correcting modifiable risk factors like sleep position or diet, then we're fighting with one arm tied behind our back (or something like that). For example, this patient has visceral obesity. Although the data on weight reduction is equivocal for GERD, the ACG guidelines still recommend weight loss where possible. She is also smoking, and the guidelines suggest quitting tobacco products based on a large cohort study indicating that smoking cessation reduces GERD symptoms by 44%.[86] She might also benefit by sleeping with a wedge pillow under her upper back and head or tilting the head of the bed to promote gravity-dependent flow of gastric contents. Remember that it's not good enough to just use a big pillow under the head; that will crank the neck but not position the esophagus and GEJ at a downward incline (**Figure 2.5**).

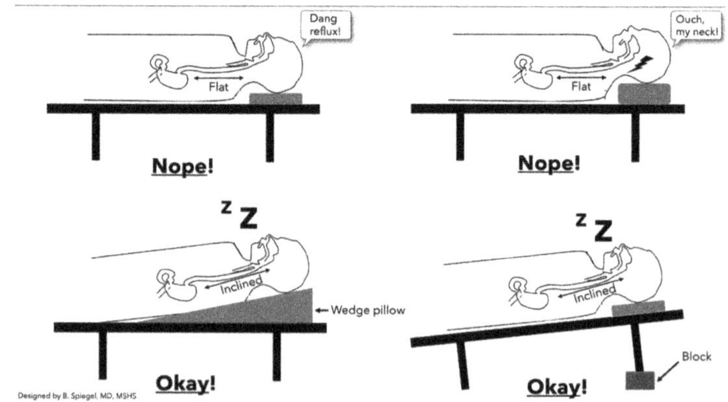

Figure 2.5. Correct vs incorrect nighttime anti-GERD positioning. (Yes, this figure is rad)

Also, patients do better when they sleep on their left side—not their right side—because that places the GEJ in a less vulnerable position for reflux. This is all pretty simple advice that can go a long way even without PPIs, although we recognize that losing weight, quitting smoking, and changing sleep habits is much easier said than done.

What about diet? The ACG guidelines recommend avoiding late night snacks, particularly within 3 hours of bedtime. That makes a lot of sense. Also, consider advising patients to avoid coffee, alcohol, chocolate, carbonated beverages, spicy food, acidic foods like citrus and tomatoes, high fat foods, and of course, peppermint (which can lower LES tone). Although evidence supporting these recommendations is weak or equivocal, dietary changes can still make a difference for some patients and it's hard to know when it will work, and when it won't. So, it's worth a try.

Okay, so you should advise this patient to lose weight, quit smoking, and eat better. That's a great start. But in this case, you're still stuck with the problem of the PPIs not working. PPIs provide complete symptom relief in 60%-70% of patients on average, with a higher response in those with confirmed erosive esophagitis (around 80% response) and lower in those with non-erosive reflux disease, or NERD (around 60% response), like with this patient. That's an impressive feat for a medication, but it also means about 30-40% of patients don't achieve complete relief despite PPI therapy.[87] **Table 2.1** lists reasons why PPIs might not be working as expected. Scan through the list, then we'll discuss the key points.

Table 2.1 *Things to consider when PPIs don't work as planned.*

Non-compliance with PPIs
Poor timing of PPIs (e.g., not taking before meals)
Underdosage of PPI—may need to double dose
Resistant to prescribed PPI—may need to switch
Non-acid reflux (e.g., bile reflux)
Hypersensitive esophagus
Concomitant disorders: • Hiatal hernia • Esophageal dysmotility • Gastroparesis • Early achalasia mimicking GERD • Eosinophilic esophagitis mimicking GERD • Reflux hypersensitivity

Start simple. Ask your patient whether they're actually taking the PPI. As doctors, we dispense all sorts of meds and assume patients take them as prescribed, but that's not always the case. In fact, it's often *not* the case. If your patient is not taking the PPI as prescribed, then use that as an opportunity to sit down together, address any questions or concerns your patient has about their disease and its treatment, and practice some good old-fashioned shared decision making. While you're at it, if your patient *is* taking their PPI, then be sure they're taking it correctly, meaning 30-60 minutes before the first meal of the day since PPIs are much more effective when used prior to proton pumps discharging their load. If your patient is having trouble adhering to the pre-meal instruction, then consider using dexlansoprazole since, unlike other PPIs, this agent's dual release mechanism and clinical benefit are not dependent on meal timing.

Dexlansoprazole is the only PPI that is not meal dependent

If your patient is taking their PPI and using it correctly, then it's worth considering whether to double the dose vs switch to another PPI. The guidelines point to one study, conducted by Fass and colleagues, that compared dose doubling vs switching to esomeprazole among patients with persistent heartburn on lansoprazole.[88] The authors found that both strategies were equally effective, with about 55% of both groups reporting a drop in symptoms. So, the jury is out on which is better. In our experience, if a patient has little-to-no benefit from once daily therapy, then it may be diminishing returns to double the dose; in that case switching to another agent might make more sense. On the other hand, if someone has a partial but incomplete response from once-daily therapy, then consider doubling the dose before switching. Notably, if you plan to switch between PPIs, remember that genetic differences in CYP2C19 metabolism can affect PPI response, so think about changing to an agent that does not rely on this enzyme for metabolism. Rabeprazole is one to consider because it does not rely on CYP2C19. On the other hand, some people knee-jerk to esomeprazole because an old meta-analysis (co-authored in part by one of your authors) found that among people with erosive esophagitis, esomeprazole has a very small but significant advantage over other PPIs.[89] But to be honest, the effect is pretty tiny, with an absolute symptom reduction of 4% vs other agents.

Also remember that different PPIs have different degrees of 24-hour pH control. When all the agents are compared to omeprazole using so-called "omeprazole equivalents," or "OEs," their relative acid-suppression potency can be ordered from highest (rabeprazole) to lowest (pantoprazole), as shown in **Table 2.2.**

Table 2.2. *Relative strength of available PPIs in relation to omeprazole equivalents (OEs).*

PPI	Relative Strength in OEs
Rabeprazole	1.82
Esomeprazole	1.60
Omeprazole	1.00
Lansoprazole	0.90
Pantoprazole	0.23

Another consideration is whether to add a histamine-2 receptor antagonist (H2RA), like famotidine or cimetidine, for patients with nocturnal GERD symptoms. When PPIs are taken in the morning, their effect dissipates as the day progresses and nighttime pH control wanes. Some have promoted use of nighttime H2RA to supplement PPI when there is an incomplete nocturnal response. The idea is that H2RAs have a rapid onset compared to PPIs and do not depend on meals, so they can help control overnight intragastric pH when added to a daily PPI regimen. However, data also indicate that this H2RA effect levels off after a month due to tachyphylaxis. In any event, the ACG guidelines do suggest adding H2RA before bedtime to help with nocturnal symptoms that are not well controlled with PPI monotherapy. That said, don't forget the sleep hygiene tips we discussed earlier!

Okay, so let's get back to this patient. She had classic GERD symptoms that did not respond to a course of once-daily PPIs. Let's assume she was taking them as prescribed and before meals. The meds still didn't work, so she was sent to upper endoscopy which was also negative (i.e., no erosive esophagitis or Barrett's mucosa). She then did reflux monitoring per ACG guidelines, which found evidence of GERD. What next?

Well, the ACG has an algorithm for how to proceed, and we'll get to it shortly. But first, when you're faced with confirmed GERD that has not responded adequately to once-daily PPIs, think about whether there might be some underlying condition that is frustrating your efforts. Maybe something else is going on to cause this bad GERD. In fact, the possibilities conveniently spell out "BAD GERD!" Check out **Figure 2.6.**

B ile reflux

A chalasia

D ysmotility of esophagus

G astroparesis

E osinophilic esophagitis

R eflux hypersensitivity

D ang hernia!

Figure 2.6. Some explanations for "BAD GERD" that doesn't respond well to once-daily PPI therapy.

Think: Could your patient have non-acidic or weakly-acidic reflux that doesn't respond to antisecretory therapy, like bile reflux? Presumably, that would have shown up on upper endoscopy but maybe you missed it at the time of the procedure. Could your patient have early achalasia or another dysmotility syndrome of the esophagus, like systemic sclerosis? If you have any question about it, then think about ordering an esophageal manometry. What about gastroparesis? As we talked about in Chapter 1, gastroparesis can present with persistent GERD. Or maybe there is underlying EoE. Again, this should have been detected on endoscopy, but maybe you missed the subtle signs of EoE or didn't get biopsies (more on EoE later in this chapter). It could be that your patient is just very sensitive to acid, or maybe has a functional esophageal condition. Unless you eradicate every drop of acid around the clock, which is not feasible even with twice-daily PPI therapy, then a patient with reflux hypersensitivity might still develop symptoms. Of course, if your patient has a hiatal hernia, then that might also undermine treatment efficacy and surgery may be warranted. We'll discuss that in a later vignette.

Let's assume you don't suspect any of the "BAD GERD" conditions. Afterall, endoscopy did not reveal signs of EoE, a hiatal hernia, or bile reflux. She doesn't have dysphagia or other symptoms of esophageal dysmotility. She does not report early satiety or postprandial nausea or vomiting, so gastroparesis is low on the list. What now? Good news, the ACG guidelines have an algorithm for this situation, shown in **Figure 2.7**.[84]

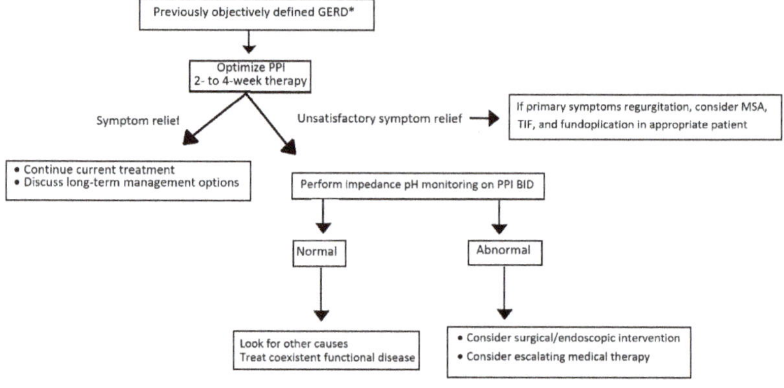

Figure 2.7. Algorithm for confirmed GERD incompletely responsive to PPIs.[84]

The next step is to "optimize" PPIs and try another course for 2-4 weeks. By "optimize," the guidelines mean trying the maneuvers we discussed before, like doubling the dose, switching to another agent like rabeprazole that doesn't rely on CYP2C19 metabolism, and if needed, adding nighttime H2RA therapy. If that works, then great; continue the treatment and discuss long-term management options.

But if optimizing PPIs doesn't work, then the guidelines say to perform impedance pH monitoring while on twice-daily PPIs. Sure, she already had reflux monitoring once, but it was *off* PPIs and performed for diagnostic purposes. In contrast, the guidance here is to repeat reflux monitoring *on* high-dose PPIs to determine whether the meds are truly blocking acid. Concurrent impedance monitoring should be performed to determine if liquid is coming into the esophagus, but it can't tell the pH of that liquid. When combined with pH-metry, the 2 modalities combined can determine whether reflux is occurring and whether the refluxate is acidic, weakly acidic, or non-acidic.

If the test is negative, meaning there is no residual evidence of acid reflux while on PPIs, then it suggests something else might be causing the symptoms beyond acid. Go back to the "BAD GERD" list to make sure you're not missing something. If you aren't, then it might be a case of functional disease, so treat that accordingly (e.g., with tricyclic antidepressants, cognitive behavioral therapy, etc.).

If the test is positive, meaning there is residual evidence of acid reflux causing symptoms despite PPIs, then it might be time to consider endoscopic or surgical interventions, particularly if regurgitation is the prominent symptom. In the next vignette, we'll discuss what the ACG guidelines say about managing persistent reflux despite optimized PPI therapy.

Case 2.3: Antireflux Procedures for GERD

A 47-year-old man complains of persistent symptoms of indigestion, heartburn, and regurgitation despite taking omeprazole 40mg every morning before breakfast. Thus, you advise that he take another dose of omeprazole 40mg in the evening. However, he notes that this provides only modest improvement. While he is on the twice daily PPI regimen, you perform an upper endoscopy with a wireless telemetry capsule attachment.

The endoscopy shows a normal appearing esophagus with a 3 cm hiatal hernia and otherwise normal stomach. The reading from the reflux monitoring reveals that the acid exposure time was 6% of the study duration. High resolution esophageal manometry is subsequently performed and reveals normal esophageal motility.

Know your guidelines!

What should you recommend next?

Case 2.3: What do the guidelines say?

Source: ACG 2021 GERD Guidelines

This patient has objective evidence of GERD that is not responding to high-dose PPIs. There is no evidence of esophageal dysmotility and no reason to suspect an undiagnosed condition contributing to recalcitrant GERD symptoms (e.g., the "BAD GERD" conditions discussed in the last vignette). This is a case of failed medical management.

In this situation, the ACG guidelines list several anti-reflux procedures for you to consider, which we'll cover in a moment. These invasive therapies are important to know about because GERD is a chronic disease, so by definition it's unlikely to just go away if first-line approaches fail. In addition, long-term PPI use has been associated with various side effects, including enteric infections, pneumonia, osteoporosis, vitamin and mineral deficiencies, kidney disease, and potentially cardiovascular (sort of everything in medicine has been blamed on PPIs at one time or another). If the PPIs ain't working, then you should stop them, not only because it's a waste of money and a burden on the patient to use PPIs indefinitely despite no benefit, but also because of their occasional adverse consequences.

The guidelines emphasize that long-term PPI use is linked with increased risk of intestinal infections, in particular, but also explain that the other associations remain debatable and not supported by randomized trials. Still, the guidelines also emphasize that we cannot fully exclude the possibility that PPIs might slightly increase the risk of these adverse events, and that further research is needed to establish causation, rather than mere association, between PPIs and their putative complications.

Okay, enough about PPIs. Let's talk about anti-reflux procedures...

But one last warning bears repeating: Before you send a patient for any anti-reflux procedure, whether surgical or endoscopic, be sure they really have GERD! Failure to respond to PPI therapy could simply mean the patient doesn't have GERD. In fact, response to PPIs is itself a strong predictor of responding to anti-reflux surgery, probably since these patients are clearly responsive to acid reduction. So, beware if a patient doesn't respond at all to PPIs; there's a good chance they don't have GERD.[90] Nonetheless, in this vignette, there is clear and objective evidence of persistent reflux despite high-dose and optimized PPI therapy, so it's reasonable to consider an anti-reflux procedure.

Anti-reflux Surgery: Laparoscopic anti-reflux surgery (LARS) has been performed since the early 1990s when it replaced open fundoplication. LARS can improve physiologic parameters of GERD by increasing LES pressure and lowering esophageal exposure time. The traditional Nissen fundoplication is a complete wrap around the esophagus, whereas partial fundoplication procedures, like the Toupet and Dor operations (**Figure 2.8**), are often preferred because they lead to fewer postoperative complications like dysphagia, gas-bloat syndrome, and inability to belch or vomit. On the other hand, there is evidence that partial fundoplication is associated with a higher rate of subsequent GERD symptoms compared to the full Nissen, so there are pros and cons with full vs partial wraps. Ultimately, choosing the best operation will depend on guidance from your surgical colleagues and their local preferences and outcomes.

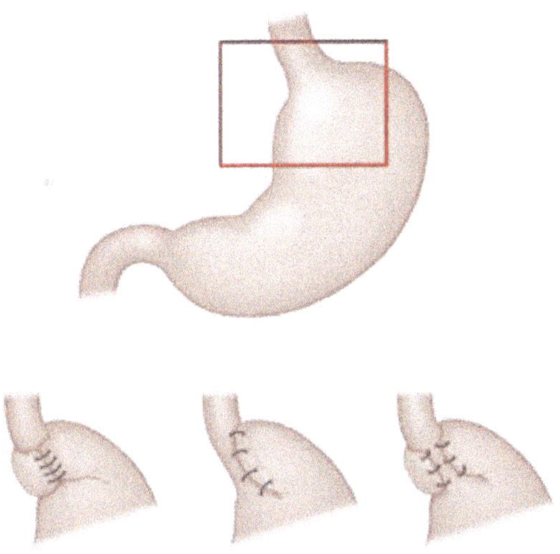

Figure 2.8. Types of anti-reflux surgery. Whereas the Nissen fundoplication is a complete wrap around the esophagus, the Dor and Toupet procedures are partial wraps.

Does LARS work? Is it better than continuing medical treatment with PPIs? This is a big topic that has been the subject of multiple competing studies. Even the meta-analyses do not fully agree on the best answer.[91,92] So, it depends. But here are some bulleted take-aways from the guidelines:

- LARS is well tolerated in most cases, but about 4% have some type of acute complication.
- Around 80% of patients can stay off PPIs long-term after LARS, but that also means about 1 in 5 go back on meds despite the operation.
- If you're sending a patient to LARS, be sure the surgeon is experienced.
- LARS might be best for those with severe reflux esopha-gitis (LA grade C or D), large hiatal hernias (like this pa-tient), and especially troublesome GERD symptoms, par-ticularly if there is regurgitation.

Magnetic Sphincter Augmentation (MSA): MSA has emerged as a viable, evidence-based alternative to LARS for certain patients with medically refractory GERD symptoms. The MSA is a ring of magnetic titanium beads that encircles the distal esophagus and bolsters the LES (**Figure 2.9**). It is not ideal for people with a large hiatal hernia and is not well-suited for managing severe esophagitis (LARS is generally preferred for both). Although MSA is easier to reverse than LARS, it has the disadvantage of being incompatible with MRI scans. The most common side effect of MSA is dysphagia, occurring in two-thirds of patients after surgery, although the risk drops to only 4% by 3 years.[93] Erosion of the beads into the esophagus is also rare, occurring in only 0.3% of cases at 4 years of follow-up.[94] Non-randomized data suggest very similar outcomes between MSA and LARS, with fewer hospital days, less dysphagia, less gas-bloat, and fewer major complications with MSA, although we are still awaiting a head-to-head randomized trial at the time of this writing. That said, MSA has been subjected to a randomized trial vs twice-daily PPIs among patients with persistent regurgitation despite once daily PPI. The study concluded that MSA was vastly superior to medical therapy, with 96% achieving control of regurgitation 1 year after surgery vs only 19% in the twice-daily PPI group.[95] As a result, the ACG guidelines strongly recommend MSA as an alternative to LARS for patients with regurgitation who fail medical management.

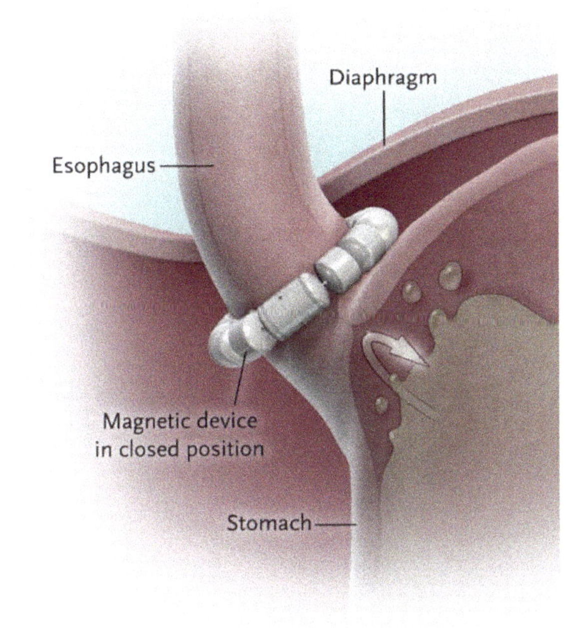

Figure 2.9. Magnetic Sphincter Augmentation. From New England Journal of Medicine, Ganz RA, Peters JH, Horgan S, et al. Esophageal Sphincter Device for Gastroesophageal Reflux Disease, 368: 719-27. Copyright ©2013 Massachusetts Medical Society. Reprinted with permission from Massachusetts Medical Society.

Roux-en-Y Gastric Bypass (RYGB): Fundoplication does not always work well in people with morbid obesity. For this reason, some consider RYGB in GERD patients with a body mass index (BMI) greater than 35 because it can simultaneously help with weight loss while also providing anti-reflux benefits. There is some controversy in this literature that goes beyond what we have time for in this brief review; check out the guidelines directly if you want to learn more. But in short, the guidelines recommend consideration of RYGB as an option to treat GERD in obese patients who are candidates for this procedures and who are willing to accepts its risks and requirements for lifestyle alterations.

Endoscopic Anti-Reflux Procedures: Not everyone with medically recalcitrant GERD wants surgery; that's where endoscopic anti-reflux procedures may play a role. The history of endotherapy for GERD goes back decades and is littered with all manner of unusual (and often dangerous) techniques to endoscopically cinch the LES. Of all the solutions proposed over the years, only one remains viable according to the ACG guidelines: transoral incisionless fundoplication, or TIF (EndoGastric Solutions; Redmond, WA). We'll talk about TIF in a second, but first, you may recall that radiofrequency treatment (Stretta; Restach, Houston, TX) is also still available as another endoscopic anti-reflux procedure. Stretta essentially burns the distal esophagus to cause swelling which is thought to tighten the esophagogastric junction. However, it remains unclear if that's really how the treatment works because a sham-controlled trial failed to show any decrease in acid exposure with Stretta. Moreover, one meta-analysis found that radiofrequency ablation did not improve quality of life or reduce the need for PPI therapy.[96] Overall, the ACG does not recommend Stretta as an alternative to medical or surgical anti-reflux therapies.

What about TIF? This procedure involves inserting a specialized endoscope that creates a flap valve at the esophagogastric junction by plicating the stomach with T-fasteners (**Figure 2.10**). Data from randomized trials indicate that TIF can improve regurgitation, although it remains unclear if the clinical benefits are durable.[97] Meta-analyses are conflicting about whether TIF can lower the need for PPI use or lower distal acid exposure.[98,99] Nonetheless, the ACG guidelines suggest considering TIF for patients with troublesome regurgitation or heartburn who do not wish to undergo anti-reflux surgery and who do not have severe reflux esophagitis (LA grade C or D) or a hiatal hernia >2cm in size.

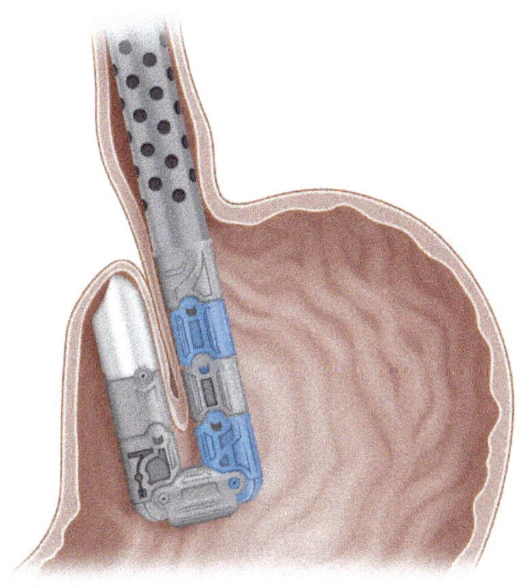

Figure 2.10. Transoral Incisionless Fundoplication.

Case 2.4: Management of Barrett's Esophagus

A 53-year-old White man living with obesity comes to your office due to reflux symptoms for the past decade. His symptoms are fairly well-controlled for the past few years with a morning dose of over-the-counter omeprazole 20 mg. He has had occasional nocturnal indigestion especially with dietary indiscretions and has found relief with use of famotidine as needed. There has been no dysphagia, early satiety, abdominal pain or nausea or vomiting. Despite his best efforts, he has been unable to lose weight or quit smoking cigars.

An upper endoscopy is performed which shows C2M5 distribution of salmon-colored mucosa in the distal esophagus. Targeted biopsies show intestinal metaplasia with goblet cells and without dysplasia.

Know your guidelines!
1. What risk factors does this patient have for Barrett's esophagus?
2. What is this patient's annualized risk of developing esophageal cancer?
3. What should you advise next?

Case 2.4: What do the guidelines say?

Source: ACG 2022 Barrett's Guidelines

Barrett's esophagus (BE) is common, so it's vital to understand how to diagnose, prognosticate, and manage this premalignant consequence of GERD. The science of BE has changed dramatically since the time your authors were GI fellows in the early 2000s. Back then, it was widely thought that patients with BE had a 10% annual risk of developing esophageal adenocarcinoma (EAC). Wow, that's scary stuff. Turns out, the true risk is much smaller than we thought. Sure, BE is premalignant in the same way that a sunburn is premalignant; both have a non-zero chance of turning into cancer, but certainly no guarantee. In both cases, the risk of malignancy is small but judicious surveillance is still needed. More on the details shortly.

But first, an homage to Dr. Nick Shaheen, the first author of the ACG BE guidelines. Dr. Shaheen has contributed massively to the GI literature, but one of our favorite studies was his elegant demonstration that BE is nowhere near as dangerous as people previously thought. Back in 2000, about the time we were fellows, Shaheen et al. published a paper demonstrating clear evidence of a "publication bias" in the literature, meaning there was a systematic absence of negative studies evaluating cancer risk in BE.[100] It's possible that journal editors were less interested in publishing negative BE studies and tended to publish large, positive studies showing that BE confers a significant risk of cancer. It turns out the literature was biased. When Shaheen and colleagues ran the numbers, they found statistical evidence of bias towards BE being more dangerous than it probably was. After accounting for the magnitude of the bias, they re-ran the numbers and estimated that the true annual EAC risk is nowhere near 10%, and maybe closer to 0.5% per year. That's a big difference! As it turns out, subsequent large-scale epidemiological studies confirmed Shaheen's downgraded estimate, and the current annual EAC

The annualized risk of EAC in Barrett's esophagus is 0.2%-0.5%

estimate is between 0.2% and 0.5% per year for BE patients without dysplasia.

Okay, let's take a step back for a moment. What is BE, anyway? The ACG guidelines define BE as *a metaplastic change of the distal esophagus, whereby the normal squamous epithelium is replaced by specialized columnar epithelium with goblet cells.*[101] The diagnosis of BE also requires at least a 1cm length of metaplastic esophageal epithelium. That's because shorter length confers a much lower risk of malignant transformation than BE exceeding 1cm, so that's an important threshold to bear in mind.

BE is most commonly a consequence of GERD and occurs in 5-12% of patients with chronic acid reflux.[102] Endoscopically, we can recognize BE as "salmon-colored" mucosa in the distal esophagus, as shown in **Figure 2.11**. However, don't proclaim that a patient has Barrett's solely because you see salmon-colored mucosa; that's a weak move. It's weak because (a) you cannot make the diagnosis of BE *unless and until a pathologist identifies intestinal metaplasia (IM) in a specimen exceeding 1cm in length obtained from the tubular esophagus* (in contrast to, say, a specimen from the gastric cardia or in a hiatal hernia), and (b) diagnosing BE prematurely can cause unneeded stress, anxiety, and even unjustifiably boost life insurance premiums.[103] Yes, that's right. Life insurance implications. There are some folks who routinely take GE junction biopsies or Z line biopsies on every EGD and incorrectly label patients with BE when IM returns on path. Remember that biopsies need to be taken at least 1 cm *above* the GE junction (more on that below). There has yet to be a significant risk found in those with IM just at the GE junction. Also, hold your horses on diagnosing BE until your pathologist makes the call. Until then, just refer to "salmon-colored mucosa" in your endoscopy report and indicate that the specimens are being sent to pathology to check for IM. If there is true BE, then you'll find out soon enough.

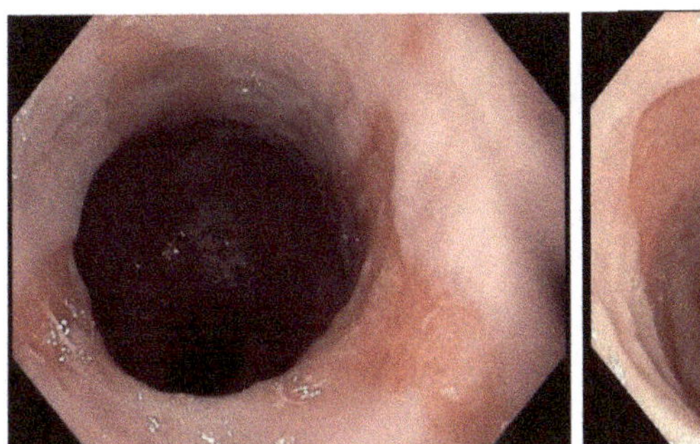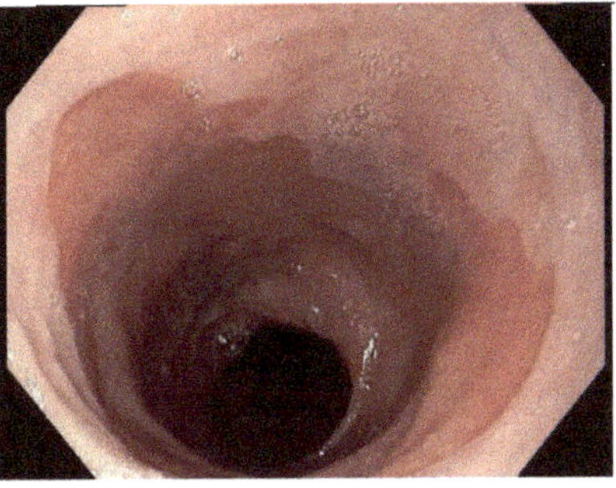

Figure 2.11. Classic salmon-colored mucosa in the distal esophagus. This is almost certainly BE, but you can't know for sure unless and until a pathologist confirms the presence of IM in the specimen. Photo from ACG image collection.

When should you screen for BE and what are its risk factors?

The patient in this vignette exhibits many of the classic BE risk factors, including:

- >5 years of GERD symptoms
- Age >50 years
- Male gender
- White race
- Tobacco usage
- Central obesity

When should you screen for BE? For starters, if you don't recall the GERD guidelines, then go back and read the last couple of vignettes to ensure you remember when endoscopy is warranted for reflux symptoms. In addition to those indications, there are certain instances when you might need to screen for BE beyond what is specified in the GERD guidelines. In particular, the ACG recommends performing a single screening endoscopy for patients with chronic GERD symptoms exceeding 5 years along with 3 or more additional risk factors for BE, including those listed in the earlier bullet points.

However, the guidelines also emphasize that general population screening for BE is not recommended or cost-effective.

The patient in this vignette is a setup for BE and screening is warranted. Endoscopy was performed and confirmed the suspicion for BE by finding salmon-colored mucosa in the esophagus that subsequently revealed IM on biopsy *but no dysplasia*. This is key, because presence vs absence of dysplasia confers a different risk of EAC, according to the data shown in **Table 2.3**.

Table 2.3. *Annual Risk of EAC Among Different Forms of BE.*

Type of BE	Annual Risk of EAC
Nondysplastic BE	0.2% to 0.5%
BE with low-grade dysplasia	0.7%
BE with high-grade dysplasia	7%

Run-of-the-mill BE without dysplasia (as seen with this patient) confers a very low risk of EAC. Patients should be clearly informed of this low risk or else they might worry about having a ticking time bomb in their esophagus. They still need surveillance, as we'll discuss shortly, but the risk of cancer is extremely low. It's worth knowing that even low-grade dysplasia confers only a small annual risk of cancer at 0.7% per year, so even having dysplastic BE is not a red alert. But, if the dysplasia is high-grade, then that's another situation as the annual cancer risk rises sharply to 7% and timely intervention is needed, as we'll soon discuss.

Best practices for performing an endoscopic "Barrett's run"

Be sure to document these 3 landmarks on any BE endo report:
• Diaphragamtic hiatus
• GEJ
• Z-Line

Let's review the best practices for describing suspected BE and performing biopsies during a "Barrett's run." A lot of people get this wrong,[104] so it's worth taking a few minutes to cover this issue in detail. When you perform an endoscopy for BE, be sure to carefully identify and document the location of the gastroesophageal junction (GEJ). Train yourself to find it. It's the spot where the end of the tubular esophagus comes in contact with the gastric folds. That may sound easy to locate in theory, but people frequently get this wrong. The esophagus also has natural folds, but those folds are different from the gastric folds. There are techniques to identify the GEJ that go beyond what we have time to describe here, but it's important to learn those techniques and make 100% sure you know how to precisely locate the GEJ. This is especially important in the presence of a hiatal hernia because it might be tricky to distinguish the GEJ from the diaphragmatic hiatus, particularly if you're over insufflating the esophagus. Moreover, the Z-line (e.g., squamocolumnar junction) is yet another landmark that may, *or may not*, be coincident with the GEJ. In fact, in BE the Z-line is decidedly *not* at the same level of the GEJ, which is why it's vital to distinguish these landmarks and describe them in your endoscopy report. Finally, if you do see salmon-colored mucosa, then describe it using the circumference and maximum extent (C&M) system, which is also called the Prague classification.[105] **Figure 2.12** shows how the BE in the current vignette would be described using the C&M system.

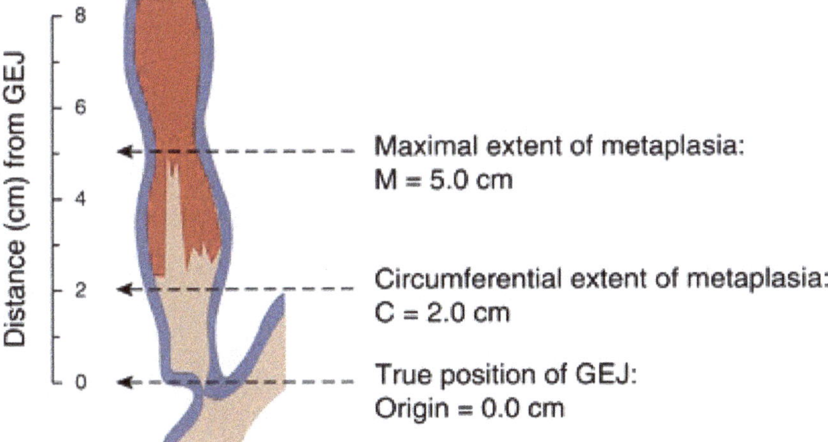

Figure 2.12. Illustration of Prague Classification for BE where C indicates circumferential extent of metaplasia and M indicates maximal extent of metaplasia. Schema shows a C2M5 segment with identification of the gastroesophageal junction (GEJ) below the squamocolumnar junction.[105]

Take at least 8 biop-
sies when screening
for BE

It's important to take a minimum of 8 biopsies when performing a Barrett's run because the diagnostic yield is higher than if you were to stop at only 4 biopsies. Ideally, you should take at least 4 biopsies per centimeter of circumferential BE, and one biopsy per centimeter along tongues of BE. Be sure to distinguish biopsies obtained in the tubular esophagus from those obtained at the cardia. Intestinal metaplasia of the cardia is common and *not* associated with EAC, in contrast to IM of the tubular esophagus. Along those lines, some people will routinely biopsy an "irregular Z-line" and then find that it contains IM.[98] *That is not BE* and should not be confused for BE.

Don't routinely
biopsy an irregular
Z-line unless there
is >1cm of proximal
extension

This is why you should not routinely biopsy an irregular Z-line unless there is more than 1cm of proximal extension. On the other hand, if you encounter a segment of BE that exceeds 3cm, then we call that "long-segment" BE.

By the way, what if the endoscopy had been negative, meaning no salmon-colored mucosa or erosive esophagitis? In that instance, the guidelines do not recommend repeating endoscopy since the chance of BE showing up later is unlikely and it is not cost-effective to keep checking for BE after the index endoscopy is negative. On the other hand, if you had found significant erosive esophagitis but no obvious BE, then you can't fully rule-out BE because the erosions might obscure the underlying lesion. In that case, the guidelines suggest treating with PPI therapy for 8-12 weeks to heal the esophagitis, and then repeating endoscopy to check for evidence of underlying BE. Finally, you might have found salmon-colored mucosa, but the biopsies came back negative for BE. In that instance, the guidelines suggest repeating upper endoscopy in 1-2 years to confirm. **Figure 2.13** summarizes the algorithm for managing salmon-colored mucosa found on endoscopy. [101]

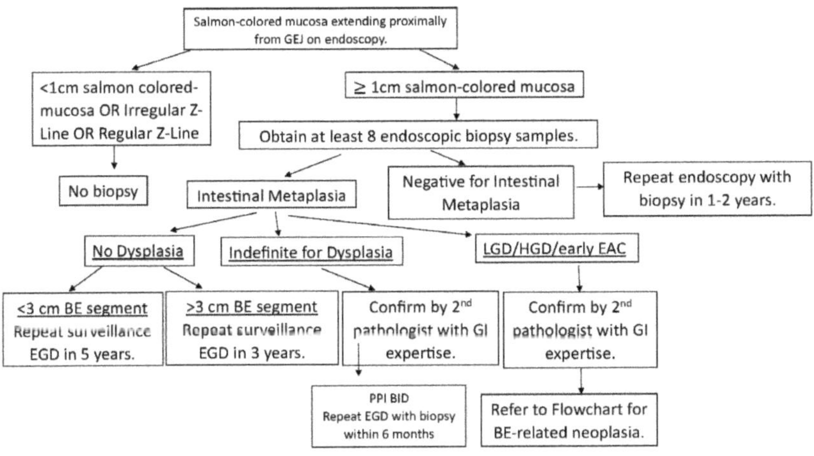

Figure 2.13. ACG algorithm for managing salmon-colored mucosa on upper endoscopy. Remember: don't biopsy an irregular Z-line with <1cm of salmon-colored mucosa! Also remember, if you do biopsy, obtain at least 8 specimens.[101]

Surveillance for confirmed BE

It is now well established from large observational studies that endoscopic surveillance of BE is associated with reduced incidence of EAC compared to patients who do not receive surveillance. Although we are still awaiting large, randomized trials of BE surveillance programs, the evidence of presumed benefit is sufficient to recommend endoscopic surveillance to eligible patients with BE. However, before starting any long-term surveillance program, patients must receive detailed counseling regarding pros and cons of surveillance, including not only the potential benefits of cancer risk reduction, but also the risks and inconvenience of repeated endoscopies, cost of the program, and small (albeit statistically significant) overall survival benefit.

Figure 2.13 outlines how to proceed once you find evidence of BE. It comes down to whether or not there is evidence of dysplasia combined with knowing the length of the BE segment. In this vignette, the patient has non-dysplastic BE extending 5cm in length. The

ACG guidelines indicate that this patient should undergo repeat surveillance in 3 years. Note, however, that if the lesion had been <3cm in length, then it would have been okay to wait 5 years before the next endoscopy. So, long segment BE should receive more frequent surveillance than shorter-segment BE, even if there is no dysplasia, because it confers a higher risk of malignant transformation.

When surveillance is performed for non-dysplastic BE, then 4-quadrant biopsies should be obtained at 2cm intervals. In contrast, when there is dysplastic BE, you should biopsy at 1cm intervals to make doubly sure you're not missing any important pathology. Also, should you ever see a mucosal abnormality (e.g., lumps, bumps, nodules, or anything that looks funny in and around the salmon-colored mucosa), those should be sampled separately and, if needed, removed with endoscopic mucosal resection (EMR). If you don't do EMR yourself, then refer the patient to someone who does.

Oh, right... do you need to use some special endoscope for BE surveillance? Does it matter, for example, if you use narrow band imaging vs high-definition white light endoscopy vs chromoendoscopy? The guidelines do not specify which to use. Just do a good job biopsying the heck out of everything regardless of which scope you're using.

What if your index procedure finds BE but the read is indefinite for dysplasia? In that case, ask a second pathologist with extensive experience in BE histopathology to render an opinion. If both pathologists are unsure, then the guidelines indicate to prescribe twice-daily PPI and repeat the endoscopy in 6 months.

If there is evidence of either low-grade dysplasia (LGD) or high-grade dysplasia (HGD), you should once again obtain a second read to confirm the diagnosis. Assuming the diagnosis is confirmed, then you should proceed according to the algorithm in **Figure 2.14**. [101]

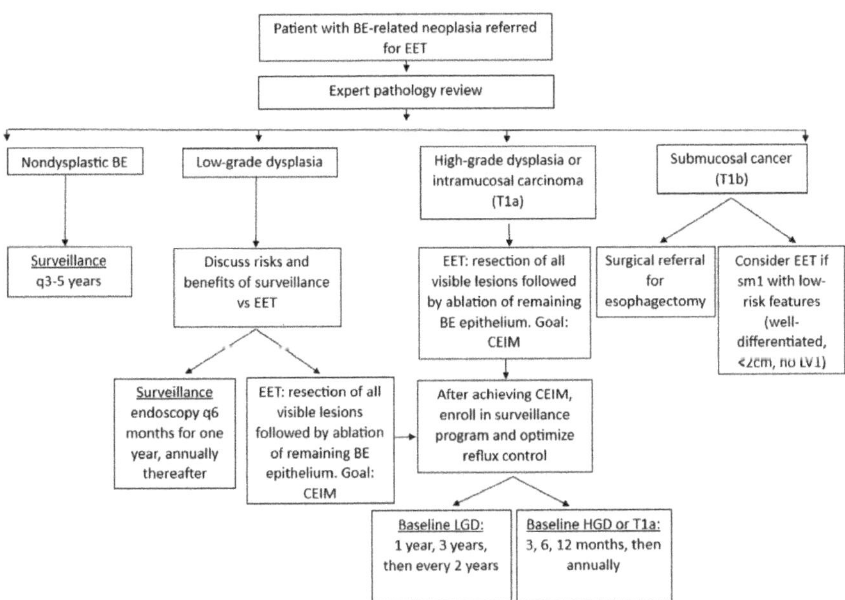

Figure 2.14. ACG algorithm for managing confirmed BE. [101]

If you encounter LGD, then the ACG guidelines recommend discussing the risks and benefits of endoscopic surveillance vs endoscopic eradication therapy, or "EET," which consists of both endoscopic removal of mucosal abnormalities through EMR combined with endoscopic radiofrequency ablation (RFA) or cryotherapy of the remaining BE epithelium. RFA is the most commonly employed ablative endotherapy based on strong evidence from randomized trials. Although older BE guidelines reserved RFA for HGD, more recent guidelines recommend this technique as an option for LGD since it is generally well tolerated and can reduce risk of EAC.

If you and your patient decide to continue surveillance in the setting of LGD, then the guideline recommends repeating endoscopy in 6 months, then again in another 6 months (i.e., 12 months following diagnosis of BE with LGD), and then annually thereafter assuming no progression to HGD or cancer. Also, if ablative endotherapy is not planned, then you should also consider treating patients with once-daily PPI therapy based on evidence that they can decrease the risk of progression to HGD and EAC by 71% based on large observational studies. Of course, it is important to remind the pa-tient that the benefits of long-term PPI therapy in this case are likely greater than the risks.

And yeah, there's more to Barrett's than that. But this will do for now. Check out the guidelines for more details.

Case 2.5: Management of EoE

A 38-year-old man presents with intermittent episodes of "food sticking in his throat" postprandially over the past several years. Previously, he drank a lot of water when this occurred and found that the food would eventually pass through. More recently however, he now finds that he has to self-induce vomiting at times to dislodge the food for relief. He has not required any emergency department visits. His only medication is rare use of calcium carbonate tablets for heartburn, which occurs after eating pizza during a late night out. Otherwise, he feels fine. There has been no weight loss, abdominal pain, or early satiety. He undergoes an EGD, which shows a ringed appearance of the esophagus. Biopsies in the proximal and distal esophagus are significant for having more than 35 eosinophils per high-power field.

Know your guidelines!

What should you recommend now?

Case 2.5: What do the guidelines say?

Source: ACG 2013 Eosinophilic Esophagitis (EoE) Guidelines

Here's another "back when we were fellows" story...

So, back when we were fellows, EoE hardly seemed to exist. Our attendings claimed they had almost never seen a case. One of us remembers scoping a patient with a food impaction, noticing mucosal rings in the esophagus (like in this vignette) and saying to his attending something like, "hey, that looks like rings, is this eosinophilic esophagitis?" No joke, the response was, "you've been reading too much! Just keep scoping!" That's what people thought about EoE back then (and what attendings thought about fellows who asked too many questions!). EoE was considered a rare disease buried deep in the textbooks and best suited for an ACG GI Jeopardy tournament, not for everyday care.

Umm, well, turns out that was wrong.

EoE started showing up everywhere. It went from a seemingly fringe condition to a prevalent disorder every fellow knows how to identify within months of starting their GI training. What happened? Were we missing cases all along? Or did something change? We're still not sure, but either way, you gotta' know EoE.

Okay, so what is EoE? For starters, the ACG guidelines distinguish EoE from esophageal eosinophilia, which is a descriptive term that does not imply any one etiology of inflammation, but rather, merely indicates the presence of eosinophils in the epithelium.[106] Esophageal eosinophilia is not synonymous with EoE—itself a unique clinicopathological disorder—although all cases of EoE are, naturally, marked by esophageal eosinophilia. That's an important distinction because there are many causes of eosinophilia in both the esophagus and other parts of the GI tract. You might favor the diagnosis esophageal eosinophilia (and eosinophilic GI disorders, or EGIDs, in general) when these risk factors are present, which conveniently spell out "EGID FAVORED."

E osinophilic esophagitis (EoE)
G ERD / graft vs host disease
I nfection / IBD (Crohn's)
D rug hypersensitivity

F ood allergens
A chalsia
V asculitis
O ther (e.g., hypereosinophilic syndromes; pollutants, celiac)
R heumatic and connective tissue diseases
E osinophilic gastroenteritis
D rug hypersensitivity (yeah, said it again because ran out of "D" causes)

Figure 2.15. The causes of esophageal eosinophilia spell out "EGID FAVORED." EoE is one of the causes, but not the only cause.

So, presence of eosinophils in the esophagus does not necessarily mean EoE. For example, GERD can cause esophageal eosinophilia. Certain drugs like NSAIDs might also cause an eosinophilic reaction through hypersensitivity, or through direct contact (e.g., pill esophagitis). Connective tissue disorder and rheumatic conditions might trigger an inflammatory response. So can certain parasitic and viral infections. And of course, it's associated with celiac disease (seems like everything is associated with celiac ;-). The list of associations is long. EoE, in contrast, is a specific cause of esophageal eosinophilia marked by "chronic, immune-mediated, esophageal disease characterized clinically by symptoms related to esophageal-predominant inflammation," as described by the ACG guidelines.[101] To diagnose EoE, the patient should have symptoms related to esophageal dysfunction (most notably, dysphagia), eosinophil-predominant inflammation on esophageal biopsy with at least 15 eos per high-power field (the patient in the vignette has 35), and no evidence of another cause of esophageal eosinophilia. Of note, the 2013 ACG guidelines are quite out of date in several ways, including its insistence that EoE cannot be diagnosed until completing a PPI trial to rule out "PPI responsive esophageal eosinophilia," which is no longer considered to be appropriate. More modern guidelines, such as the American Gastroenterological Association (AGA) guidelines on EoE,[107] have removed the PPI trial from the diagnostic criteria of EoE. We eagerly await an updated ACG EoE guideline to reflect this important advance. In any event, you should obtain at least 2-4 biopsies from both the proximal and distal esophagus when screening for EoE, and should also obtain biopsies from the antrum and/or duodenum to rule out a broader EGID if there are any gastric or small intestinal symptoms or endoscopic abnormalities in those areas.

The ACG guidelines emphasize that a "typical" EoE patient has a history of atopy and/or asthma, is male (male to female ratio is 3:1), and presents with first esophageal symptoms either in childhood or during the third or fourth decade of life. Although it can occur in any racial or ethnic group, EoE also tends to occur more commonly among non-Hispanic Whites.

There are several characteristic features of EoE on endoscopy, including mucosal edema, esophageal rings (also called "trachealization"), white exudates, longitudinal furrows (which can easily tear if you're not careful), and a small caliber "feline" lumen with strictures. These conveniently spell out "EREFS" (**E**dema, **R**ings, **E**xudates, **F**urrows, **S**trictures), an easy way to remember the 5 classic endoscopic features of EoE that also form basis of the standard EREFS scoring system for EoE.[108]

Speaking of "trachealization," by the way, one of your authors unceremoniously intubated a patient's trachea when he was a first-year fellow and immediately thought he was seeing EoE only to quickly arrive upon the carina. Not good. Thankfully, the patient did just fine, but the supervising attending certainly did not do fine. Suffice it to say, that misstep has never been repeated.

Anyway...

Figure 2.16 shows a typical appearance of a ringed esophagus. Bear in mind that rings are neither pathognomonic nor required to diagnose EoE. In fact, the endoscopy occasionally will be normal in patients with EoE,[109] so you should maintain a low threshold to biopsy if your pre-test likelihood is high enough.

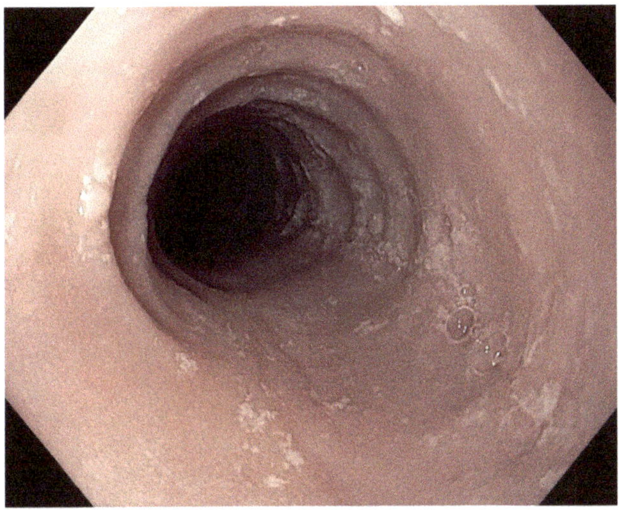

Figure 2.16. Typical appearance of ringed esophagus. Image source: Evan Dellon, MD.

Okay, so let's suppose you see an esophagus like the one in Figure 2.16, which is similar to the findings described in the vignette. Your antennae should be up for EoE, but you can't know for sure that it is EoE yet. Since you've read the ACG guidelines on EoE (or at least, read this book), you will know to obtain *at least* 2-4 biopsies in both the distal and proximal esophagus. If the biopsies return evidence of >15 eos per high power field, then you know EoE is likely, but even then, be sure to rule out the other "EGID FAVORED" diagnoses. **Figure 2.17** outlines the approach you should follow as recommended by the AGA guidelines[107] (the 2013 ACG guideline is no longer accurate, so we need to use AGA guidelines here until the ACG guideline update is complete).

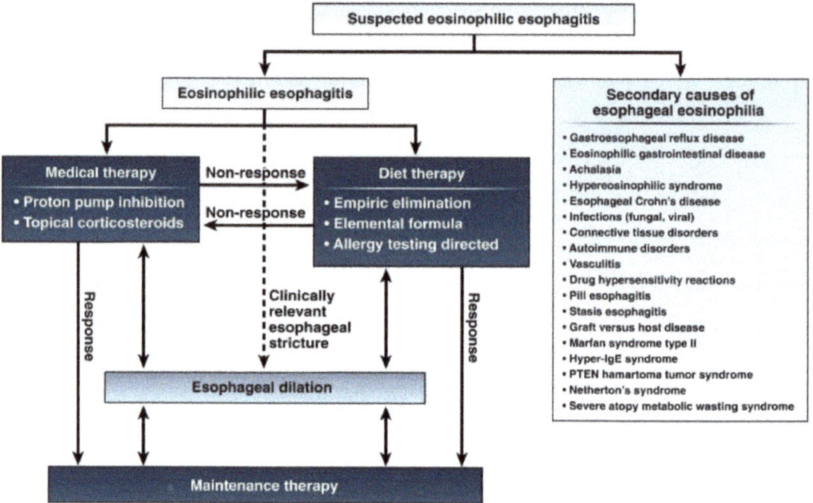

Figure 2.17 Algorithm for evaluating and treating suspected EoE. Reprinted from Gastroenterology, Vol 158, American Gastroenterology Association. Treatment of Eosinophilic Esophagitis (EoE) Clinical Decision Support Tool. Page 1787, Copyright 2020, with permission from Elsevier.

After you discover eosinophils in the esophageal mucosa, you should next consider the differential diagnosis we previously discussed. If there are no competing explanations, and assuming the eosinophilia is isolated to the esophagus, then you can diagnose EoE and consider a few therapeutic options, including medical therapy, diet therapy, and/or endoscopic therapy with dilation (if there is a clinically relevant esophageal stricture).

EoE Treatments

Proton Pump Inhibitors: Both the 2013 ACG and more recent 2020 AGA guidelines recommend starting with PPIs as first line medical therapy. Meta-analysis of studies examining the effect of PPIs in EoE indicate an overall histological response rate and remission rate of 61% and 51%, respectively.[110] That's pretty good, although it should be noted that the studies are quite heterogenous, making it hard to draw firm conclusions about the benefits of PPIs. Nonetheless, it's generally a good idea to start with PPIs before steroids since they are so well tolerated and associated with a reasonable response in many patients.

Topical steroids: Assuming PPIs don't work, then the usual next step is to try topical corticosteroids.[111,112] Consider using either fluticasone or budesonide in daily divided doses. These meds come in either multi-dose inhalers (MDIs) or as a nebulized solution. The steroid must be swallowed, not inhaled. It should ideally be mixed into a viscous suspension with a flavoring agent (e.g., honey or chocolate syrup) to cut down on the bitter taste of the steroid. We've seen patients get confused or even misinformed by pharmacy instructions that fail to emphasize the correct mode of administration, leading patients to inhale the steroids and then return without feeling any better. Also, don't forget that candidiasis is a notable side effect of all topical steroids.

Leukotriene inhibitors: Nope. Although useful for asthma, these agents have not panned out for EoE and do not maintain steroid-induced remission.[113]

Dupilumab: At the time of this writing, the most recent ACG EoE guidelines were still dated 2013, which we've already noted is pretty ancient. There have been important updates in EoE treatment, and we will revise this text once the newest guidelines are published. In the meantime, we felt it was important to emphasize a more recent advance in EoE management that was not mentioned in the 2013 guidelines: monoclonal antibodies to block the interleukin-4 (IL-4) receptor. Dupilumab is an injectable IL-4 receptor alpha antagonist that reduces proinflammatory cytokines, chemokines, and immunoglobin E. A randomized trial revealed that dupilumab leads to histological remission in 60% of patients, compared to only 5% of controls while improving the frequency and severity of dysphagia.[114] The most common adverse reactions include injection site reaction, upper respiratory tract infections, arthralgia, and herpes viral infections. So, just know about this one. We'll update once the new ACG EoE guidelines are published.

Dietary therapy: We've been talking about medical therapies so far, but dietary therapy can often be effective for EoE and, at least for some patients, may be the preferred initial strategy, as suggested by Figure 2.17. There are 3 diets covered by the guidelines. The first is to simply eliminate all food allergens by consuming an elemental diet. The second approach is to employ skin prick allergy testing to guide a targeted elimination diet. And the third is the famous "6 food elimination diet," which involves, you guessed it, eliminating the top 6 food groups known to trigger EoE: milk, egg, soy, wheat, nuts, and seafood. One of your authors has a lot of trouble remembering this list (the other seems to remember everything), so he just

N uts

E ggs

W heat

S oy / **S** eafood

M ilk

A nd...

N uts again
(because there are a bunch of tree nut triggers)

Figure 2.18. Components of Six-Food Elimination Diet for EoE.

imagines that Anderson Cooper, the CNN "newsman," is having a heck of a time trying to swallow his food (which is maybe just ridiculous enough to work as a memory aid, shown in **Figure 2.18**.)

The elemental diet is considered to be the most effective, but that is not an easy diet to follow and is costly. Skin prick testing is also costly compared to an empiric 6-food elimination. Moreover, targeted diets based on skin prick testing don't work much better than empiric diets, so they are no longer recommended (in contrast to the ACG 2013 guidelines, which are outdated on this point). Simply eliminating cow's milk alone may be the optimal initial dietary strategy. When selecting the best diet for your patient, find out more about their preferences and resources and consider collaborating with a dietician and/or allergist. Be sure that the patient follows the diet for at least 4-8 weeks before any reintroduction period and follow the patient clinically and with endoscopic surveillance to see if there is a histological improvement. For more details on diet, check out the guidelines which provide a lot more information than we'll cover here.

Case 2.6: Management of Achalasia

48-year-old woman has a long history of heartburn with indigestion, which has been more pronounced at night over the past 2 decades. Her symptoms have progressed over time with initial improvement on omeprazole 40 mg daily but now has not responded to a twice daily dosage increase. In addition, she has developed dysphagia of solids and liquids over the past couple of years despite following a soft vegetarian diet. She spends almost one hour to eat her meals and has lost 13 pounds in the past 4 months. Despite sleeping on a wedge pillow, she still has awakened with regurgitation and retrosternal discomfort.

Know your guidelines!

What is the next most appropriate step?

Case 2.6: What do the guidelines say?

Source: ACG 2020 Achalasia Guidelines

Let's start with a fun fact: the word "achalasia" is derived from the Greek root "khalan," which means "to relax," and of course the prefix "a-" means "not" or "without." So, achalasia literally means *no relaxation*. And that's spot on, because the *sine qua non* of achalasia is failed LES relaxation with swallowing. But as we'll learn shortly, the story gets a little more complicated because there's another LES relaxation problem that *isn't* achalasia. More on that in a bit (in the meantime, think about it now and see if you know what we're talking about).

As seen in this vignette, achalasia typically presents with progressive dysphagia to solid and liquids, often with heartburn and chest pain along with weight loss or nutritional deficiencies. Also evident in this case is that the peak onset for achalasia is between the ages of 30 and 60 years old. Because heartburn is a common symptom of achalasia, the diagnosis can sometimes be confused with GERD in the earlier stages before dysphagia becomes prominent. That's why the ACG guidelines recommend that patients with PPI-unresponsive GERD be evaluated for achalasia, as discussed earlier in the book.

We'll get back to the clinical aspects of achalasia in a moment, but we first need to discuss what causes this condition. You may recall from studying GI physiology that LES function reflects a balance between excitatory and inhibitory neurons. During a normal swallow, the contracted LES appropriately loosens, allowing food to pass from the esophagus into the stomach. This is enabled by activation of inhibitory nerves, particularly those that release vasoactive inhibitory peptide (VIP) and nitric oxide (NO). In contrast, the excitatory neurons release acetylcholine (ACh), which keeps the LES cinched, blocking acid and other gastric contents from moving proximally into the esophagus. However, when there is selective loss of VIP and NO secreting neurons the net effect is unopposed muscular contraction from ACh-secreting excitatory neurons, leading to a tight LES that is unable to relax (*i.e.*, a-chala-sia). That gets to the crux of achalasia: it results from selective loss of inhibitory neurons in the myenteric plexus of the distal esoph-agus and LES.[115]

Okay, with that brief review of pathogenesis, let's work through the management guidelines for achalasia. **Figure 2.19** shows the ACG algorithm.[115]

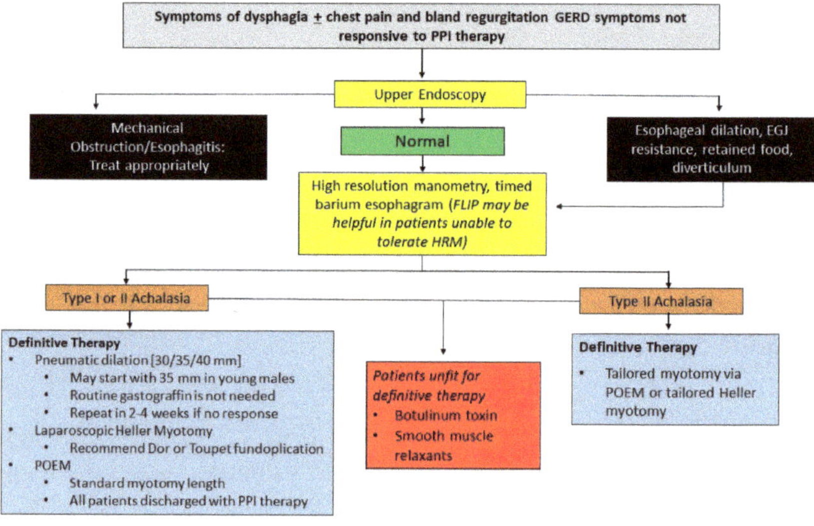

Figure 2.19. ACG Diagnostic and Treatment Algorithm for Suspected Achalasia.[115]

The algorithm starts with a patient who has dysphagia, chest pain, and bland regurgitation that has not responded to PPI therapy. If you see a patient like this, then it's time for an upper endosco-py. Although endoscopy is not the gold standard for diagnosing achalasia, there are several endoscopic clues that should make you think of the diagnosis, especially evidence of retained saliva with a puckered gastroesophageal junction that's hard to traverse despite normal amounts of pressure (**Figure 2.20**). Retained food, a distal esophageal diverticulum, and a dilated esophagus are other findings that should make you think of achalasia.

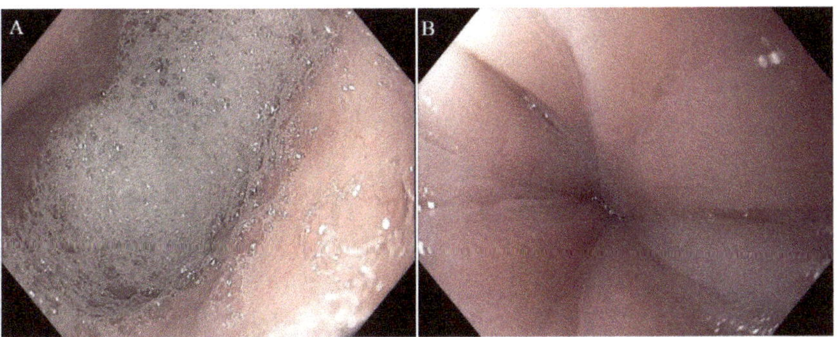

Figure 2.20. Endoscopic Appearance of Achalasia. (a) Foamy retained saliva. (b) "puckering" of the gastroesophageal junction.[115]

Another important reason to perform endoscopy is to exclude pseudoachalsia, in which a tumor at the gastroesophageal junction erodes into the LES, leading to preferential destruction of inhibitory neurons and unopposed annular contraction.

Although performed less frequently than before, patients with dysphagia may undergo a barium esophagram prior to endoscopy. You'll probably remember the 'ole "bird's beak" esophagus that shows up with barium, marked by a tight distal esophagus with proximal dilation, as shown in **Figure 2.21**, below. If you squint, it looks like a hummingbird hanging upside down from a branch.

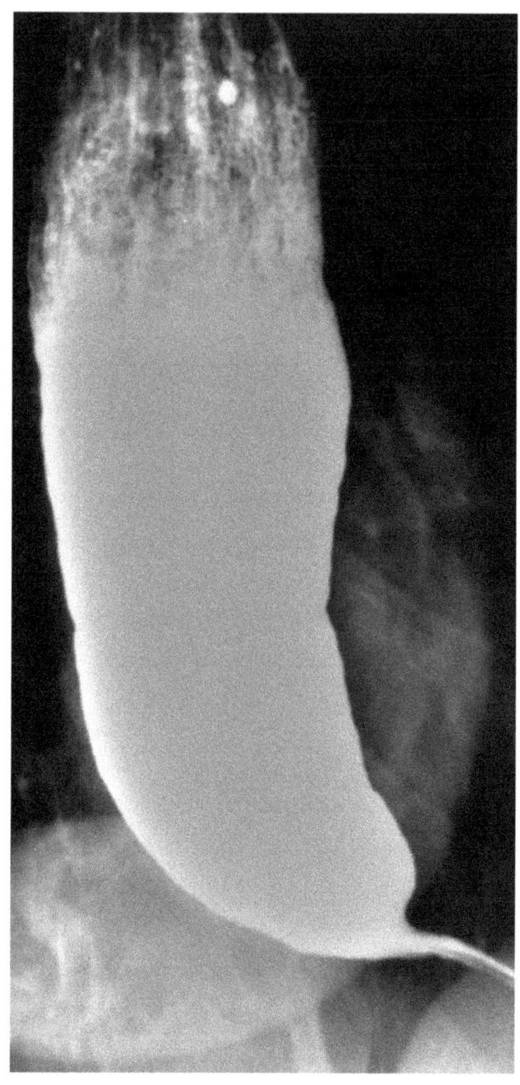

Figure 2.21. Barium Swallow Showing Classic "Bird Beak" Esophagus with Proximal Dilation. Source: ACG Achalasia Guidelines.[115]

The gold standard diagnosis of achalasia requires esophageal high-resolution manometry (HRM). We won't have time to review all the ins-and-outs of HRM so we suggest you check out other sources for the details. Here, we'll point out the key HRM features of achalasia and assume you've seen HRM heatmaps before and know something about how they're read.

Okay, to set up the discussion around manometry and continue following the algorithm in **Figure 2.19**, we need to introduce the Chicago Classification of achalasia.[116] While we're at it, we also need to distinguish achalasia from esophago-gastric junction (EGJ) outflow obstruction. And yes, EGJ outflow obstruction was the other condition we were alluding to at the beginning of this discussion. **Figure 2.22** lays it all out.

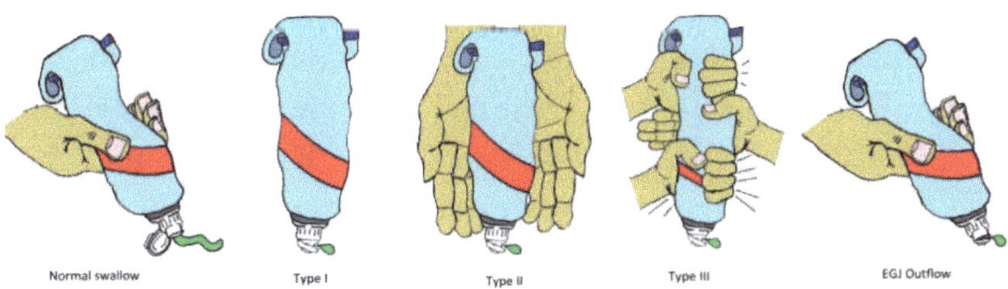

Figure 2.22. Distinguishing a normal swallow from the 3 forms of achalasia and contrasting with EGJ outflow obstruction. Credit to Dr. Jonathan Gotfried, MD, who conceived this very creative memory aid.

You may recall that we used a toothpaste analogy last chapter when discussing defecatory disorders (see Figure 1.7). Here, we're using the analogy again, this time with respect to the esophagus. Under normal circumstances, when you swallow a food bolus there is peristalsis driving the material towards the LES. But also—and this is critical—there is appropriate *relaxation* of the LES to allow effortless transit of the bolus into the stomach. Figure 2.22 depicts a normal swallow as squeezing the toothpaste while opening the cap, thus allowing the paste to squirt out the bottom. EGJ outflow obstruction, in contrast, occurs when there is appropriate peristalsis but no LES relaxation as shown in the right panel of Figure 2.22.

> EGJ outflow obstruction has tight LES but *normal* peristalsis

Achalasia is different from both normal swallowing and EGJ outflow obstruction *because there is no peristalsis*. As with EGJ outflow obstruction, the LES does not appropriately relax with achalasia, but remember that EGJ outflow has normal peristalsis, whereas achalasia does not.

The Chicago Classification describes 3 forms of achalasia which are, unsurprisingly, called Type I, Type II, and Type III.[115] Type I is what we used to think of as "classic" achalasia before the Chicago Classification. Type I is characterized by aperistalsis with pan-esophageal pressurization that does not exceed 30 mm Hg. Type II, in contrast, does have esophageal pressurization above 30 mm Hg, but the pressurization is not spastic or obliterative. Figure 2.22 depicts Type II as lightly cupping the tube but not squeezing it too hard. Type III goes a step further with lumen obliterating yet aperistaltic contractions, depicted as haphazard grabbing of the tube. We used to call this "vigorous achalasia" before the Chicago Classification renamed it Type III achalasia.

So, what's the most common type of achalasia? It would be convenient if the answer were Type I, but alas, it isn't. Type II achalasia is most common, accounting for 50-70% of cases. Type I is second most common, accounting for 20-40% of cases. Finally, Type III is the rarest form, bringing up the rear with ~5% of cases.

Now that we've set it up, we can study the 3 classic HRM pictures of Types I-III achalasia, as shown in **Figure 2.23.** [115]

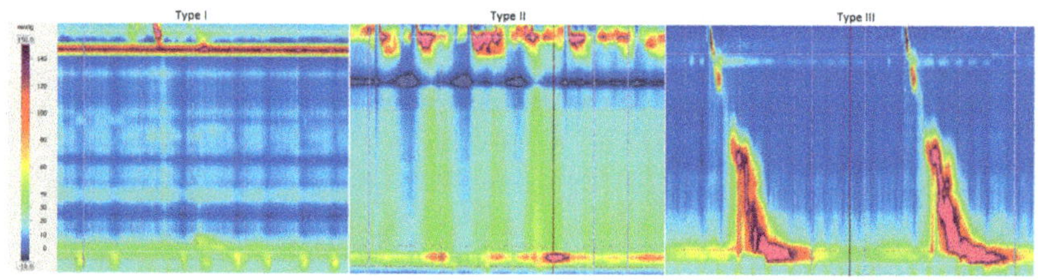

Figure 2.23. HRM of Types I-III achalasia. Source: ACG Achalasia Guidelines.[115]

You'll notice in all 3 panels of Figure 2.23 that there's a solid green and yellow bar at the bottom of the tracing; that's the LES pressure zone, and at no point does it break in any of the images, even with wet swallows. We like to imagine the HRM as a topographical map depicting water and land from above, where the blue part is water and the other color parts are land masses of different altitudes (red=highest altitude). Normally, the blue "water" (so to speak) would breach the "dam" at the bottom and break through the bar, but with achalasia (and EGJ outflow obstruction), the water does not cross the dam. The blue does not break through like it does in **Figure 2.24** showing a normal swallow.

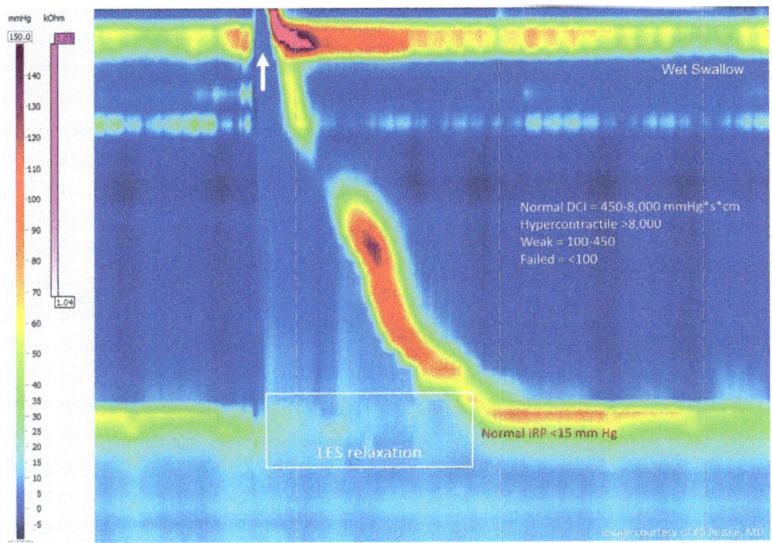

Figure 2.24. HRM of a normal swallow. Note the "ocean" breaks thorough the "dam" at the bottom, indicating LES relaxation which is not seen with achalasia. Image source of Ali Rezaei, MD.

So, returning to Figure 2.23, all 3 types of achalasia are marked by a solid green bar at the bottom, indicating lack of LES relaxation. In Type I, there is no pressurization; it just looks like the ocean without any land within the sea. In Type II, there is some pressurization, which appears like a solid green column cutting through the blue space. You'll notice that the column is vertical, not diagonal as seen with the normal peristaltic swallow in Figure 2.22. In Type III, there's a red-hot, vertical bar indicating high pressure, obliterative contractions, like a tall mountain range cutting through the water. But remember, just because there are contractions does not mean there is peristalsis; Type III has *a*peristaltic yet intense contractions.

Okay, pop quiz:

- What's the most common type of achalasia?
- Which type of achalasia has <30 mm Hg of pressurization?
- Which type of achalasia is least common?
- Which type of achalasia has obliterative peristalsis?

Got it? So, what did you say? Don't just read this sentence and jump straight to the answers. See if you can go back and get the answers before you read on. Okay, we're going to type a few lines of text here to keep you reading before you get to the answers. And… here come the answers. The most common type? That's Type II. The type with <30 mm Hg of pressurization? Type I. Least common? Type III. The type with obliterative peristalsis? Uhm…*none* of them. None have peristalsis (that was a trick question).

Before we move onto therapy, a quick word about FLIP, which stands for *functional lumen imaging probe*. FLIP is an FDA-approved high-resolution impedance system that measures the cross-sectional area and distensibility of the esophagus. The data from FLIP converts into a geometric model of the esophagus that offers information about motor function and EGJ opening dynamics. Research indicates that FLIP is useful to diagnose achalasia and is highly correlated with HRM results.[117] Because manometry can be very difficult for some patients to tolerate, the ACG guidelines recommend FLIP as an alternative since it can be administered during endoscopy under sedation.

Okay, let's move on to treatment. Here's a key point to remember: the treatment of Type I and II achalasia is different from the treatment for Type III. That's the whole point of the Chicago Classification, because the different forms of achalasia have different prognoses and treatment protocols. Figure 2.1 makes that clear since there's a fork in the algorithm separating out Types I/II from Type III.

The ACG guidelines distinguish "definitive therapies" for achalasia from, well, less definitive therapies. Less definitive therapies include oral medications like nitrates, calcium channel blockers, anticholinergics, and sildenafil, all of which aim to loosen the LES. They don't work great, so we'll leave it at that. Instead, the definitive therapies for Type I and II achalasia are focused on disrupting the LES musculature. Here are the definitive therapies for Types I and II achalasia:

Pneumatic Dilation (PD): PD involves blowing up a big balloon in the LES and stretching the muscles apart. These balloons are bigger than the usual dilations you might perform for an esophageal stricture where the sizes range from around 5mm to 20mm diameter balloons. That's small fries compared to what's needed for achalasia, where you'll need a 30mm minimum sized balloon inflated under fluoroscopy. Because these are big-time balloons, you need to always be prepared to bring the patient to surgery if things go sideways, which means *it's best to not even consider a PD for achalasia in someone who isn't fit for surgery*. The technical details of PD are beyond what we'll cover here, but in short, most start with 30mm diameter balloons, followed later by serial dilations to 35mm and 40mm. The only exception is achalasia in young males, who tend to fare well with the 35mm balloon at initial dilation. PD provides good-to-excellent relief in 50% to 93% of patients, which is a fairly wide range and dependent, in part, on the training and skill of the operator. Predictors of PD success include older age (>45 years), female sex, narrow (nondilated) esophagus, and LES pressure after PD of <10mm Hg, indicating adequate tearing of the LES musculature.[115] Esophageal perforation occurs in 2% of patients on average.[118] Because perforation can be serious, some endoscopists will perform routine gastrograffin esophagram after PD to check for early signs of a perforation, but the ACG guidelines do not recommend this as routine practice because it's generally low yield. Finally, post-procedural GERD occurs in up to 35% of patients after PD. When that happens, it should be treated aggressively with PPIs to reduce stricturing, which is the last thing a patient with achalasia needs (well, nobody goes around asking for a stricture, but you know what we mean).

Surgical Myotomy: The goal of surgical myotomy is to divide the muscle fibers of the LES to facilitate food passage into the stomach. Data reveal that the laparoscopic approach is preferred over laparotomy and thoracotomy approaches.[115] Surgical myotomy yields a clinical response rate ranging from 60% to 94%, with better responses for Type I and II achalasia than Type III, which is always the tougher form to treat. Post-myotomy GERD is a common problem affecting nearly one-third of patients, but if myotomy is followed by a surgical fundoplication, then the incidence of GERD falls to only around 9%. For this reason, the ACG guidelines recommend combining myotomy with fundoplication to control distal esophageal acid exposure. Both the Dor or Toupet fundoplication are considered equivalent and acceptable per the guidelines.

Peroral Endoscopic Myotomy (POEM): The POEM procedure uses an endoscopic approach to form a submucosal tunnel along the distal body of the esophagus, eventually accessing the circular muscle fibers of the LES where a myotomy is performed. Success rates are high, with over 90% of patients achieving clinical benefits.[119] POEM is often used for the recalcitrant Type III achalasia where the obstructive contractility is addressed, in part, by the esophageal tunneling. In contrast, Types I and II respond well to LES-focused treatments and do not usually require POEM to achieve clinical benefit. In addition, the length of the myotomy can be tailored with POEM to address the spastic segment as determined by HRM or FLIP, which is another reason this is the preferred initial therapy for most people with Type III achalasia, although Heller myotomy can also be used for these patients (see **Figure 2.17** again for details). As with other achalasia treatments, post-procedural GERD is also a problem with POEM and requires aggressive PPI treatment to avoid esophagitis and peptic strictures.

Botulinum Toxin Injection: Direct injection of botulinum into the LES is inferior to myotomy and is reserved for patients who are unfit for more definitive therapy because they are not surgical candidates. For that reason, it is not considered a first-line therapy for any form of achalasia, except for those who cannot tolerate definitive therapy (e.g., think of an elderly achalasia patient with multiple comorbidities).

One last bit: How best to monitor patients after they've been treated? There are various approaches, but the ACG guidelines recommend using a timed barium esophagram (TBE) to determine whether there is evidence of bolus retention or EGJ obstruction. The details of TBE are beyond what we'll cover here, but check out the guidelines if you want more information. Also, know that the risk of esophageal squamous carcinoma is higher in achalasia than controls. This is thought to result from ineffective esophageal motility with stasis and inflammation contributing to dysplasia and carcinoma. Nonetheless, data do not support routine endoscopic surveillance as it's unclear this practice actually improves survival. The guidelines ultimate recommend against routine endoscopic surveillance and call for more research.

We'll end with this handy table summarizing the differences between Types I-III achalasia.

Table 2.4. *Chicago Classification of Achalasia*

Chicago Classification type	Old Name	Manometric Features	Treatment Success Rates	Definitive Treatment
Type I	Classic achalasia	No esophageal pressurization >30mm Hg	Intermediate chance of responding to treatment (44%)	1.Pneumatic dilation 2. Heller myotomy 3. Standard length Poem
Type II	N/A	Simultaneous isobaric pressurization >30mm Hg across entire esophagus	Most likely to respond to treatments (80%); "early form" of achalasia	
Type III	Vigorous/ spastic	Lumen-obliterating contractions or spasams	Least likely to respond to treatments (9%)	1. Tailored myotomy via POEM 2. Tailored Heller myotomy

Esophagus Guidelines Quiz

1. What duration of PPI therapy is recommended before performing upper endoscopy for a patient with GERD and no alarm features?

    a) 4 weeks
    b) 6 weeks
    c) 8 weeks
    d) 10 weeks
    e) 12 weeks

2. Which of the following statements about long-term use of PPIs in GERD patients is true?

    a) PPIs should be discontinued after 4-8 weeks of therapy
    b) Long-term PPI use is associated with an increased risk of gastric cancer
    c) PPIs are not effective for maintenance therapy in GERD
    d) PPIs should be prescribed at the lowest effective dose for symptoms

3. According to the ACG guidelines, which of the following is NOT a recommended lifestyle modification for the management of GERD?

    a) Weight loss (if overweight or obese)
    b) Elevating the head of the bed
    c) Avoiding food triggers
    d) Regular physical exercise
    e) Sleeping on left side

4. For how long should PPIs be discontinued before performing diagnostic upper endoscopy for GERD?

    a) 1-3 weeks
    b) 2-4 weeks
    c) 3-5 weeks
    d) 4-6 weeks
    e) No need to discontinue PPIs before diagnostic upper endoscopy.

5. Which of the following patients has definitive "GERD" as defined by the ACG guidelines?

   a) LA class A erosive esophagitis without Barrett's esophagus
   b) LA class A erosive esophagitis with <3 cm segment of Barrett's esophagus
   c) <3 cm segment of Barrett's esophagus without erosive esophagitis
   d) LA class B erosive esophagitis without Barrett's esophagus
   e) B and D both have GERD

6. Pathologic acid reflux is defined by an acid exposure time (AET) exceeding which of the following thresholds?

   a) 2%
   b) 4%
   c) 6%
   d) 8%
   e) 10%

7. A patient with GERD is found to have a circumferential segment of biopsy-proven Barrett's esophagus extending from 38cm to 40cm. The GEJ is located at 40cm. There is a tongue of Barrett's mucosa extending from 34cm to 38cm. Which of the following describes this patient's "C&M" classification?

   a) C0M2
   b) C2M0
   c) C4M2
   d) C2M2
   e) C2M6

8. Which of the following is true about reflux monitoring?

   a) Wireless telemetry should be employed for 48-96 hours.
   b) Transnasal telemetry should be employed for 48 hours.
   c) Transnasal telemetry is not capable of discriminating among acidic, weakly acidic, and non-acidic reflux.
   d) Reflux monitoring should be conducted while on PPIs when attempting to diagnose GERD.

9. Which of the following is true about use of PPIs for GERD?

a) PPIs provide complete symptom relief in around 50% of patients, on average.

b) There is no difference in symptom relief with PPIs between GERD patients with vs without erosive esophagitis.

c) Unlike other PPIs, the effect of dexlansoprazole is not pH sensitive.

d) Among patients on lansoprazole with partial relief of GERD symptoms, switching to esomeprazole is superior to doubling the dose of lansoprazole.

e) There is no difference between the available PPIs in terms of their ability to heal erosive esophagitis.

10. Which of the following PPIs has the greatest relative strength in terms of "omeprazole equivalents"?

a) Pantoprazole
b) Lansoprazole
c) Esomeprazole
d) Rabeprazole

11. Which of the following PPIs is not metabolized by CYP2C19?

a) Pantoprazole
b) Lansoprazole
c) Esomeprazole
d) Rabeprazole
e) Omeprazole

12. Of all the adverse consequences of PPIs that have been described, which of the following is supported by randomized controlled trial data?

a) Pneumonia
b) Renal disease
c) Osteoporosis
d) Vitamin deficiencies
e) Enteric infection

13. Which of the following is true about laparoscopic anti-reflux surgery (LARS)?

    a) Over 90% of patients stay off PPIs after LARS.
    b) LARS is most effective for patients with LA class A and B esophagitis.
    c) Compared to a full Nissen fundoplication, partial wraps like Toupet and Dor operations have a lower risk of post operative GERD.
    d) Acute complications are uncommon after LARS, occurring in 4% of patients.

14. Which of the following is true about magnetic sphincter augmentation (MSA)?

    a) MSA is incompatible with MRI scanners.
    b) It is best suited for patients with a large hiatal hernia.
    c) Dysphagia is rare following MSA.
    d) Nonrandomized data indicate that LARS is more effective than MSA.
    e) Randomized data indicate that MSA is equivalent to BID PPI therapy

15. Which of the following is true about endoscopic anti-reflux procedures?

    a) Radiofrequency ablation of the lower esophageal sphincter (Stretta procedure) decreases acid exposure in the distal esophagus.
    b) Among all the endoscopic anti-reflux procedures, only transoral incisionless fundoplication (TIF) is recommended by the ACG.
    c) Data indicate that use of Stretta reduces the need for PPI therapy.
    d) Meta-analysis definitively shows that TIF can lower the need for PPI therapy.
    e) TIF is most effective for patients with severe reflux esophagitis (LA grade C or D)

16. Which of the following describes presence of a "publication bias," as was discovered in the Barrett's esophagus literature?

    a) Relatively few large and negative studies
    b) Disproportionate number of small, positive studies
    c) Relatively few small, negative studies
    d) Disproportionate number of large, negative studies

17. Which of the following most closely estimates the annual incidence of esophageal adenocarcinoma among patients with non-dysplastic Barrett's' esophagus?

    a) 0.02%
    b) 0.2%
    c) 2%
    d) 5%
    e) 10%

18. What is the minimum length of metaplastic esophageal epithelium required in order to diagnose Barrett's esophagus?

    a) 0.5 cm
    b) 1.0 cm
    c) 1.5 cm
    d) 2.0 cm
    e) 2.5 cm

19. A patient with heartburn undergoes EGD. There is an irregular Z-line within 1 cm of the GEJ but no other abnormalities. Biopsy of the Z-line reveals intestinal metaplasia. When should the next surveillance endoscopy be performed?

    a) 6 months
    b) 12 months
    c) 3 years
    d) 5 years
    e) No surveillance is indicated.

20. Which of the following is <u>not</u> a risk factor for Barrett's esophagus?

    a) >5 years of GERD symptoms
    b) White race
    c) Age >45 years
    d) Tobacco usage
    e) Central obesity

21. Which of the following most closely estimates the annual incidence of esophageal adenocarcinoma among patients with high-grade Barrett's' esophagus?

    a) 1%
    b) 3%
    c) 5%
    d) 7%
    e) 9%

22. A minimum of how many biopsies is recommended when performing a "Barrett's run" during endoscopy?

    a) 2
    b) 4
    c) 6
    d) 8
    e) 10

23. Endoscopy reveals a 2 cm segment of nondysplastic Barrett's esophagus. When should the next surveillance endoscopy be performed?

    a) 1 year
    b) 2 years
    c) 3 years
    d) 4 years
    e) 5 years

24. A patient with longstanding GERD symptoms undergoes EGD which reveals 3 cm of salmon-colored mucosa along with LA class B erosive esophagitis. Biopsies do not reveal intestinal metaplasia. What is the next most appropriate step?

   a) Treat with PPI therapy for 8-12 weeks, do not repeat endoscopy.
   b) Treat with PPI for 4-6 weeks and then repeat endoscopy.
   c) Treat with PPI for 8-12 weeks and then repeat endoscopy.
   d) Treat with PPI therapy on demand for GERD symptom management.

25. Endoscopy reveals a 5 cm segment of Barrett's esophagus. When should the next surveillance endoscopy be performed?

   a) 1 year
   b) 2 years
   c) 3 years
   d) 4 years
   e) 5 years

26. Endoscopy reveals 3 cm of Barrett's mucosa that is deemed "indefinite" for dysplasia by 2 pathologists. In addition to PPI therapy, when should EGD be repeated?

   a) 3 months
   b) 6 months
   c) 12 months
   d) 24 months

27. A patient with heartburn undergoes EGD. There is an irregular Z-line within 1 cm of the GEJ but no other abnormalities. Biopsy of the Z-line reveals intestinal metaplasia. When should the next surveillance endoscopy be performed?

   a) 6 months
   b) 12 months
   c) 3 years
   d) 5 years
   e) No surveillance is indicated.

28. A patient is found to have Barrett's esophagus with low-grade dysplasia and opts to continue surveillance with PPI therapy rather than use endoscopic eradication therapy. Which of the following surveillance schedules is most appropriate?

a) Repeat endoscopy every 3 months indefinitely.
b) Repeat endoscopy in 3 months, then again in another 3 months, then every 6 months indefinitely
c) Repeat endoscopy in 6 months, then in another 6 months, then annually
d) Repeat endoscopy annually.

29. Which of the following conditions is <u>not</u> associated with esophageal eosinophilia?

a) Ehlers Danlos Syndrome
b) Celiac sprue
c) Crohn disease
d) Achalasia
e) Graft vs host disease

30. To diagnose eosinophilic esophagitis, a patient should have symptoms related to esophageal dysfunction and at least how many eosinophils per high-power field on esophageal biopsy?

a) 10
b) 15
c) 20
d) 25
e) 30

31. Which of the following is the most appropriate first-line therapy for a patient with dysphagia found to have esophageal eosinophilia with >15 eos per high powered field?

a) Systemic steroid
b) Leukotriene inhibitor
c) Dupilumab
d) Proton pump inhibitor

32. Dupilumab blocks which of the following interleukin (IL) receptors?

a) IL-1
b) IL-2
c) IL-3
d) IL-4
e) IL-5

33. Which of the following is <u>not</u> part of the 6-food elimination diet for EoE?

a) Gluten
b) Wheat
c) Eggs
d) Shellfish
e) Tree nuts

34. The HRM tracing, below, is most consistent with which of the following diagnoses?

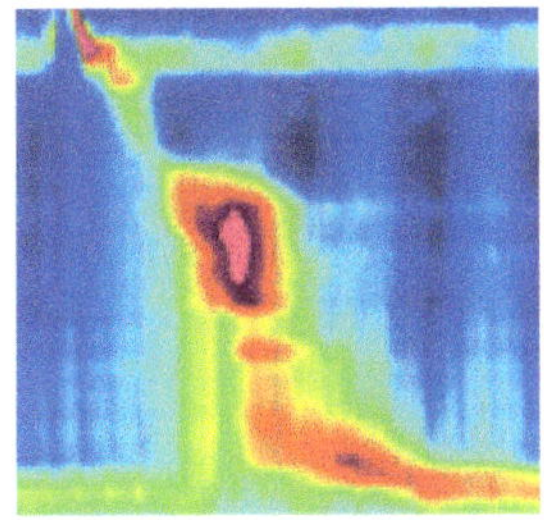

a) Type I achalasia
b) Type II achalasia
c) Type III achalasia
d) EGJ outflow obstruction
e) Jackhammer esophagus

35. The HRM tracing, below, is most consistent with which of the following diagnoses?

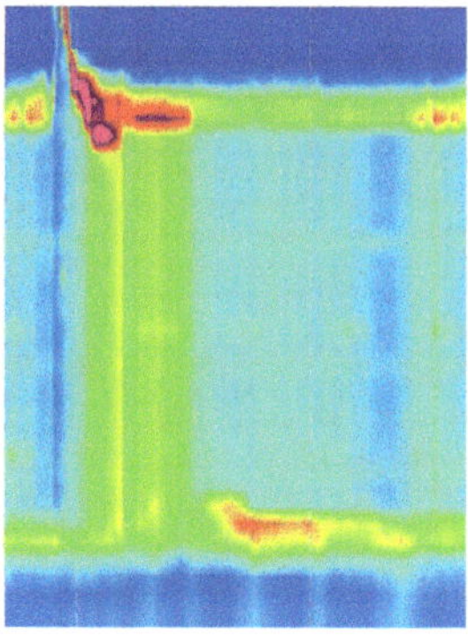

a) Type I achalasia
b) Type II achalasia
c) Type III achalasia
d) EGJ outflow obstruction
e) Systemic sclerosis

36. The HRM tracing, below, is most consistent with which of the following diagnoses?

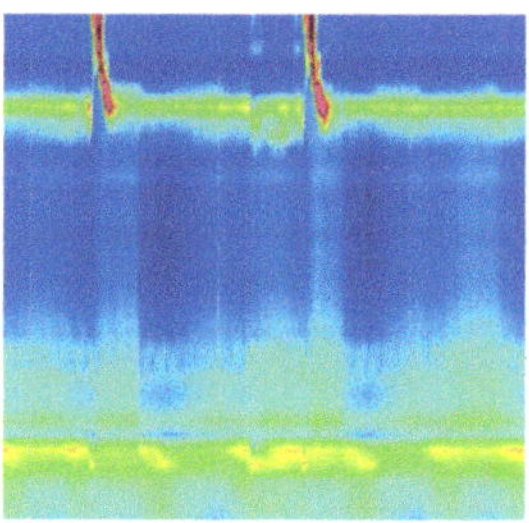

a) Type I achalasia
b) Type II achalasia
c) Type III achalasia
d) EGJ outflow obstruction
e) Jackhammer esophagus

37. The HRM tracing, below, is most consistent with which of the following diagnoses?

    a) Type I achalasia
    b) Type II achalasia
    c) Type III achalasia
    d) EGJ outflow obstruction
    e) Polymyositis

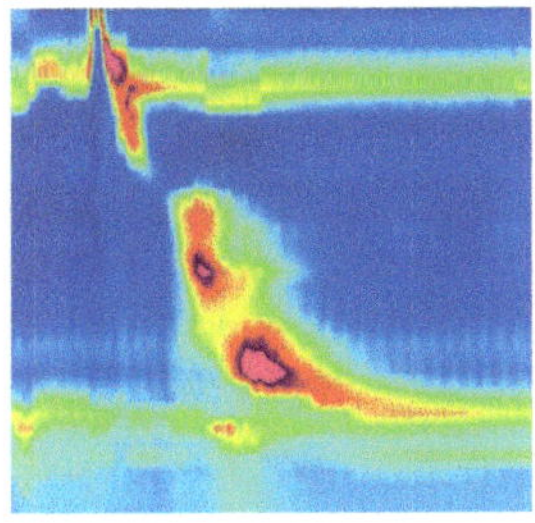

38. Which of the following is the most common type of achalasia?

    a) Type I achalasia
    b) Type II achalasia
    c) Type III achalasia
    d) Pseudoachalasia

39. Which of the following is marked by obliterative peristalsis?

    a) Type I achalasia
    b) Type II achalasia
    c) Type III achalasia
    d) EGJ outflow obstruction
    e) Jackhammer esophagus

40. Which of the following is not a predictor of success for pneumatic dilation in achalasia?

    a) Age $\geq$ 45 years
    b) Male sex
    c) Narrow esophageal caliber
    d) LES pressure after PD < 10mm Hg

Esophagus Guidelines Quiz Answers

1.	C	21.	D
2.	D	22.	D
3.	D	23.	E
4.	B	24.	C
5.	D	25.	C
6.	B	26.	B
7.	E	27.	E
8.	A	28.	C
9.	C	29.	A
10.	D	30.	B
11.	D	31.	D
12.	E	32.	D
13.	D	33.	A
14.	A	34.	C
15.	B	35.	B
16.	C	36.	A
17.	B	37.	D
18.	B	38.	B
19.	E	39.	E
20.	C	40.	B

CHAPTER THREE

LUMPS AND BUMPS

Polyp and Cancer Prevention Guidelines

Lumps and bumps. We see a lot of those in gastroenterology. In fact, we're like honorary dermatologists, only we're *endo*-dermatologists. It just happens that we're concerned with lumps and bumps on the inside, not on the outside. And just like dermatologists, we need to know how to identify epithelial lesions, how to remove them, and whether and how to follow-up to prevent cancer.

In this chapter, we'll discuss the full range of GI lumps and bumps, with a special focus on colon polyps and colorectal cancer (CRC) screening, surveillance, and prevention—the "bread and butter" of gastroenterology. We'll also address GI polyposis syndromes, hereditary GI cancer syndromes, gastric premalignant conditions, and submucosal masses. Let's start with the basic CRC screening guidelines, then we'll branch out from there.

Case 3.1: Noninvasive Stool Testing for CRC Screening

A 46-year-old woman Caucasian woman in good health with no family history of cancer is sent to you by her primary care physician for discussion about CRC screening. She takes no medications and has no significant past medical history. She feels well and has no change in bowel habits, abdominal pain, weight loss, bleeding, or anemia. She explains that she is hesitant to undergo colonoscopy but is willing to do less invasive forms of CRC screening, including stool tests. She wants your opinion about the role of stool testing and asks about the accuracy and outcomes of stool testing vs colonoscopy for CRC screening.

Know your guidelines!

1. How sensitive and specific is fecal immunochemical testing (FIT) vs colonoscopy?
2. What is the comparative effectiveness of FIT testing vs colonoscopy for clinical outcomes including cancer detection and mortality?
3. How sensitive and specific is multitarget stool DNA testing vs colonoscopy?

Case 3.1: What do the guidelines say?

Sources: ACG 2021 CRC Screening Guidelines; ACG 2017 FIT Guidelines

Colonoscopy remains the gold standard for CRC screening. However, there's an oft-quoted truism about screening: "the best test is the one that gets done." Even though gastroenterologists generally support colonoscopy as the best test for screening,

"best" can mean different things to different people and many patients (most, in fact) prefer *noninvasive* stool testing over invasive colonoscopy. You might think that more patients would select colonoscopy if they fully understood that a positive stool test still requires colonoscopy but, alas, that's not the case. In fact, one of your authors participated in a study showing that even knowing that stool testing is imperfect, and even knowing that a positive test still mandates full colonoscopy, *most patients still prefer stool testing.*[120] So, it's important to understand the details on noninvasive stool testing. And it's vital that, despite our general bias towards colonoscopy, we employ shared decision making to arrive at a suitable option for each patient. Our job is to make sure to "get 'er' done," so to speak! This patient needs *some* form of screening to help reduce her 4% mortality risk for CRC. She is in good health and otherwise has a predicted long survival.

This vignette sets up the problem well and illustrates a scenario that plays out almost daily in the GI clinic. It's common that patients are willing to do CRC screening but less willing to do colonoscopy. This patient has very reasonable questions about noninvasive screening tests, their pros and cons, and the overall outcomes of stool-based screening. To answer these questions, we turn to the ACG guidelines on FIT, which includes a discussion about multi-target stool DNA (mt-sDNA) testing.[121]

As a quick review, recall that FIT is different from the old guaiac-based tests of yesteryear. The old tests did not directly measure human hemoglobin, but instead detected peroxidase activity. Since human hemoglobin is a peroxidase catalyst, guaiac-based tests indirectly detect human hemoglobin but also falsely alert in the presence of other peroxidase catalysts, including a variety of iron-containing foods. In contrast, FIT tests are a *direct* measure of human hemoglobin and therefore reduce the risk of false positive testing, improving specificity. Importantly, FIT remains approved by the US Preventive Services Task Force as a viable CRC screening test, whereas guaiac-based tests are not. As an aside, FIT was never intended to help emergency department providers and hospitalists distinguish normal stool from melena or hematochezia. It's not a screening test for GI bleeding, it's a screening test for CRC! (okay, pet peeve off our chests now ;-)

So, how accurate is FIT when compared to the gold standard of colonoscopy (bearing in mind that colonoscopy is itself a tarnished gold standard)? Meta-analysis reveals a pooled sensitivity and specificity of 79% and 94%, respectively, for FIT's ability to detect cancer.[122] It's positive predictive value maxes out at 7.8% across studies, meaning that if a patient has a positive test, then there is a roughly 8% chance of underlying cancer. As expected, the sensitivity of FIT drops to around 20%-30% when predicting advanced adenomas rather than cancer, although its specificity remains over 90% for advanced lesions. Because FIT has a relatively low accuracy, it must be repeated annually to be effective at detecting advanced adenomas and/or CRC on a timely basis. Of course, positive tests require colonoscopy follow-up.

What can we tell this patient about the overall effectiveness of FIT vs colonoscopy? We are still awaiting results of the definitive randomized trial on this topic, which is years in the making and, as of this writing, still a few years out from final results. Stay tuned. In the meantime, one study found no difference in CRC detection between a FIT and colonoscopy, likely because participation was much higher in the FIT arm (34% vs 25%).[123] In per protocol analysis, there was a nonsignificant trend towards improved CRC detection in those randomized to the colonoscopy arm. But overall, it's hard to say at this time that one strategy is clearly superior over the other; more data are eagerly awaited.

What about mt-sDNA testing? It's important to know that the leading mt-sDNA test is actually a combination of both FIT and DNA testing. When using a one-time test, the sensitivity and specificity of mt-sDNA testing for CRC is 92% and 87%, respectively, compared to colonoscopy.[124] That means DNA testing is more sensitive than FIT, but slightly less specific Keep in mind that mt-sDNA is only FDA-approved for screening *average* risk patients.

Patients often become very concerned when they get a positive mt-sDNA test. There is understandable concern since 4% of patients with a positive test harbor colon cancer. In fact, about half of patients with a positive test will have adenomatous colon polyps. But that also means that there are a lot of false positive results. So, what do you do when an asymptomatic patient with a positive mt-sDNA test subsequently gets a normal high-quality colonoscopy? Is the colonoscopy itself falsely negative? This has been studied and can perhaps make you and your patient relax a little. In a study with over a combined 1,000 patients with a positive mt-sDNA test and negative colonoscopy, there were only 8 aerodigestive cancers discovered at 4 years of follow-up.[125] This incidence rate was similar to the general population and also similar to those who had a negative mt-sDNA test. Another trial also confirmed these findings.[126] That means no additional testing is needed after a normal colonoscopy in the setting of a positive mt-sDNA test. No need for an upper endoscopy, abdominal CT, or repeating the colonoscopy earlier than otherwise indicated. As long as a *high-quality* colonoscopy was performed, you can go back to routine average risk screening recommendations. That is, repeat the mt-sDNA test in 3 years or another colonoscopy in 10 years. There will certainly be more DNA tests in the future, but they haven't been adequately studied to be recommended in the guidelines at this point.

Case 3.2: Colon Cancer Screening

A 67-year-old new patient is referred for a screening colonoscopy by his primary care physician without medical records. He reports that over the past 2 years he has had gradually increasing dyspnea. He now gets short of breath when he walks to the bathroom and subsequently increases his continuous oxygen that he receives by nasal cannula with any minimal exertional activity. He is still smoking a pack of cigarettes daily but hopes to quit. He notes that he takes "a lot of water pills" to keep the swelling down in his legs and sees a cardiologist and pulmonologist every month or 2. While taking this history, you note that he has labored breathing and ask him about it. He responds, "Today is one of my better days. It's usually a lot worse." There have been no warning signs or symptoms or diagnostic tests to suggest that he is at increased risk for CRC. He wants to know how to set up the colonoscopy.

Know your guidelines!
1. Would you proceed with colonoscopy?
2. Is there another colon cancer screening test that you would recommend for him?
3. What is the age limit for a screening colonoscopy?

Case 3.2: What do the guidelines say?

Source: ACG 2021 CRC Screening Guidelines

The guidelines indicate that this patient should not undergo a screening colonoscopy.[127] In fact, he should not get screened for CRC at all. In this case, you don't have medical records to review, but it illustrates that taking a good history is of utmost importance. It is even more crucial than the physical examination, which was also absent in this example. At any rate, this patient has too many active cardiopulmonary problems to consider CRC screening, which provides limited benefits in this case. He could be harmed by CRC screening and would likely not be eligible for abdominal surgery if CRC were discovered. The risks outweigh the benefits for him.

What if his primary care provider screened him and then obtained a positive stool-based test and it came back positive? Would you propose that this patient pursue the potential risks associated with a colonoscopy? This is where shared decision making is the key to guiding the best outcomes. There is no single best answer; you need to look at the situation holistically and rationally, and then work with your patient to arrive at a mutually agreeable decision.

A related question: at what age do you stop routine CRC screening? In general, screening benefits are obtained at least 7-10 years down the road.[128] So, you don't want to be screening those who are not likely to live much past that time span. We know to screen healthy adults ages 45 to 75; however, the US Preventive Services Task Force (USPSTF) recommends that screening over age 75 needs to be individualized with attention paid to the patient's overall health and screening history. Moreover, those over 86 years old should not be screened due to competing causes of mortality at that age.[129] Our aging population warrants careful consideration without knee-jerk testing for everyone.

Now that you know what the guidelines say about average risk CRC screening, let's turn to those with a family history. It can get a little tricky. Say that you are seeing another patient whose father had CRC diagnosed at age 53. When should this patient obtain a screening colonoscopy in the absence of any warning signs or symptoms? The ACG guidelines recommend starting screening at age 40, or 10 years prior to the affected relative, whichever is earlier. Since age 40 is earlier than age 43 (10 years before age 53), this hypothetical patient with a family history should obtain a screening colonoscopy at age 40 with interval colonoscopies every 5 years if negative assuming the first-degree relative was diagnosed under age 60. If the patient had 2 or more first-degree relatives at any age with CRC, then the interval is also every 5 years.

What about another patient whose mother had CRC at age 68? Here, the guidelines also recommend starting at age 40 (since age 40 is earlier than 10 years prior to the affected first-degree relative). If the colonoscopy is negative in a patient with first-degree relative over age 60, future screening follows the average risk profile with colonoscopy every 10 years.

Okay, what about screening someone with a family history of colon polyps? Not all polyps are created equal. The guidelines count a family history of a first-degree relative with an "advanced polyp" as equivalent to the risk of having a first-degree relative with CRC.[130] For example, one trial demonstrated that siblings with an advanced adenoma had an 11.5% prevalence of having an advanced adenoma versus 2.5% among siblings without a family history of advanced adenomas.[131] By the way, when the guidelines mention "advanced polyp," they are not talking about small hyperplastic polyps in the rectosigmoid. Nor small tubular adenomas. But they do include serrated polyps since there is more and more data pointing towards serrated polyps being a significant precursor lesion to colorectal cancer (more on that in a later vignette). Look at the **Table 3.1**, below, for the advanced polyp criteria.

Table 3.1. *Advanced polyp criteria.*

Adenomatous polyps	Serrated polyps
Adenomas ≥10 mm	Sessile serrated lesions ≥10 mm
Adenomas with villous histology	Sessile serrated lesions with dysplasia
Adenomas with high-grade dysplasia	Traditional serrated adenoma

The guidelines apply the same screening recommendations for patients with a first-degree relative with CRC as they do for those with a first-degree relative with an advanced polyp; they do not distinguish these patients. Thus, you can just substitute family history of a first-degree relative with an advanced polyp as family history of a first-degree relative with CRC into the screening guideline recommendations.

Finally, don't forget that performing a high-quality colonoscopy is of paramount importance. We will briefly review quality measures in relation to colonoscopy later in this chapter. Suffice it to say that a high-quality colonoscopy is absolutely necessary to properly screen for CRC.

Case 3.3: Colonoscopy Follow-Up

You are seeing a 55-year-old woman who has relocated due to a transition in employment and has moved into your area. She wants to know when she should get her next colonoscopy. She has no family history of CRC or colon polyps. She is feeling well and reports no change in bowel habits and no rectal bleeding, anemia, or weight loss. You review the records that she has brought in and note that she had a colonoscopy with cecal intubation and a good bowel preparation 5 years ago. The colonoscopy was remarkable for complete removal of a 7 mm tubular adenoma from the transverse colon and a 5 mm tubular adenoma from the sigmoid colon. She has been worried that she waited too long to get another colonoscopy.

Know your guidelines!

Is she overdue for colonoscopy?

Case 3.3: What do the guidelines say?

Source: U.S Multi-Society Task Force on Colorectal Cancer 2020 Guidelines on Follow-Up After Colonoscopy and Polypectomy

Thankfully, you can reassure her that she is not behind schedule or overdue for surveillance colonoscopy. In fact, this patient can wait a couple of years to get her surveillance colonoscopy. It used to be that we would do a surveillance examination within 5 years; however, it has been shown that those with low-risk findings (1-2 nonadvanced adenomas <10 mm) on initial colonoscopy don't have much of an increased risk of metachronous colon cancer. A large study with nearly 16,000 patients found that there was no significant colon cancer risk between patients with nonadvanced adenomas compared with no adenoma (RR, 1.2 [95% CI 0.8-1.7]; P = 0.30) over a median of 13 years of follow-up. However, those with advanced adenoma were at increased colon cancer mortality risk compared with the no adenoma group (RR, 2.6 [95% CI, 1.2-5.7], P = 0.01).[132]

Again, it's important to reiterate what constitutes advanced or high-risk adenoma features on baseline colonoscopy, which we discussed in the last vignette. It also makes sense that if one has multiple (3 or more) adenomas removed on a single colonoscopy, then your risk for metachronous colon cancer in the future is increased. A meta-analysis with over 10,000 patients found that there was a small increase in metachronous advanced neoplasia over a 5-year time horizon in those with 1 or 2 small adenomas (4.9%) versus those with a normal baseline colonoscopy (3.3%). Moreover, those with high-risk adenoma on baseline examination had a 17% risk after subsequent colonoscopy in 5 years.[133] This is shown in **Figure 3.1.**

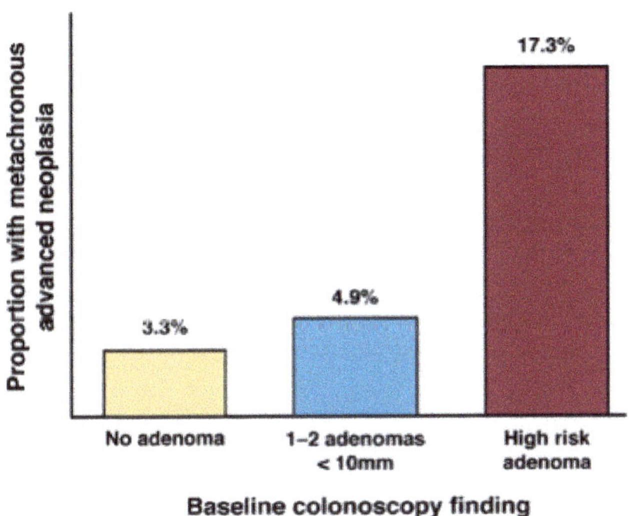

Figure 3.1 Risk for metachronous advanced neoplasia 5 years after baseline colonoscopy.[135]

Therefore, the surveillance interval can be shorter depending on the baseline examination findings.

What if she had a baseline normal colonoscopy without any polyps detected? Should she even get screened again in 10 years? The answer for now is yes. Rescreening those 10 years after a baseline screening colonoscopy has been studied and shown to confer some benefit. In fact, repeat screening is estimated to reduce colon cancers from 31.3 per 1000 persons to 7.7 cases per 1000 persons.[134] Thus, repeat screening recommendations for colonoscopy has remained at 10 years after a normal examination.

When providing future surveillance recommendations, it is vital that a high-quality index colonoscopy is performed. These features are noted below in **Table 3.2**.

Surveillance guidelines assume a high-quality colonoscopy was performed at baseline

Table 3.2 *High-Quality Colonoscopy Criteria.*

Complete examination to the cecum
Withdrawal time >6 minutes
Bowel preparation adequate to identify polyps >5 mm
Colonoscopist has adequate adenoma detection rate
Complete polyp resection

The various strategies for follow-up of adenomatous colon polyps have been updated in the recommendations by the United States Multi-Society Task Force (USMSTF) on colorectal cancer, which are summarized in **Table 3.3** below.[135]

Table 3.3 *USMSTF Adenoma Surveillance Recommendations for Average-Risk Patients.[134]*

Finding	Surveillance Interval
Normal	10 years
1-2 tubular adenomas < 10 mm	7-10 years
3-4 tubular adenomas < 10 mm	3-5 years
5-10 tubular adenomas < 10 mm	3 years
Adenoma $\geq$10 mm	3 years
Adenoma with villous histology	3 years
Adenoma with high-grade dysplasia	3 years
10 or more adenomas on one exam	1 year
Piecemeal resection of adenoma $\geq$20 mm	6 months

Case 3.4: Sessile Serrated Polyp

An asymptomatic 47-year-old man at average risk for CRC undergoes his initial screening colonoscopy. During scope withdrawal, the lesion in **Figure 3.2,** below, is noted in the ascending colon and completely resected with a cold snare. Pathology reveals a 7 mm sessile serrated polyp with clear resection margins. Afterwards, the patient sends you a portal message asking when he should plan his next colonoscopy. He also wants to know what lifestyle modifications can help reduce his risk for getting more polyps.

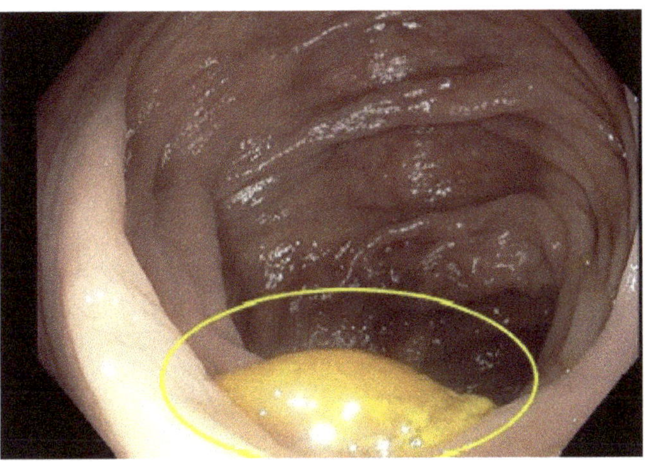

Figure 3.2. Colon polyp. Image source: Brennan Spiegel, MD, MSHS

Know your guidelines!

1. When should this patient next undergo surveillance colonoscopy for his 7 mm sessile serrated adenoma?
2. Would the answer to #1 be different if this were a 7 mm tubular adenoma?
3. What would you do if this had been a 20 mm sessile serrated polyp that was removed in piecemeal fashion?
4. Speaking of serrated polyps, when should you suspect serrated polyposis syndrome?
5. What lifestyle modifications can reduce his risk for metachronous neoplasia?

Case 3.4: What do the guidelines say?

Source: U.S Multi-Society Task Force on CRC 2020 Guidelines on Follow-Up After Colonoscopy and Polypectomy

He should have his next colonoscopy in 5-10 years.[134] This recommendation is slightly different for sessile serrated polyps (SSPs) vs tubular adenomas (TAs). If this had been a single, sub-centimeter TA, then the next colonoscopy would be in 7-10 years. **Figure 3.3** demonstrates the surveillance recommendations depending on the findings from colonoscopy. [135] Keep this image tattooed on the back of your hand (actually, don't do that, because it seems to change every few years ;-)

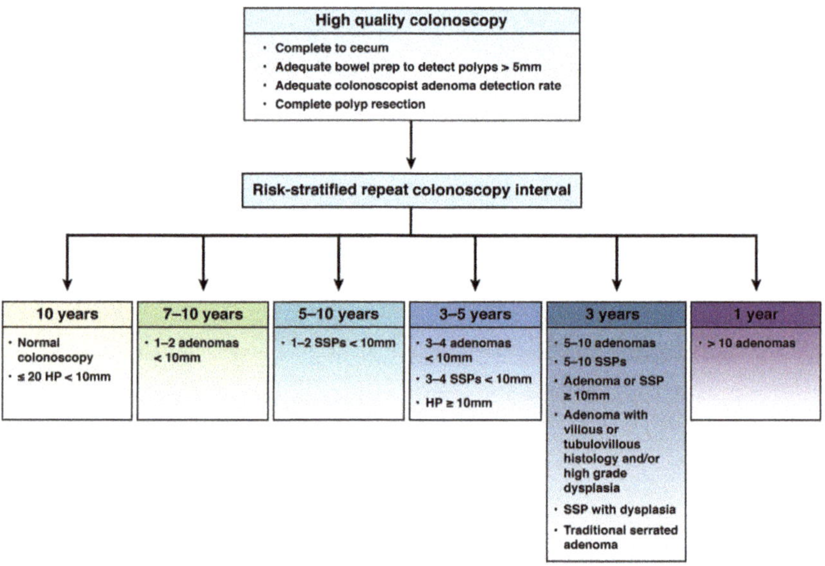

Figure 3.3 USMSTF Recommendations for Follow-Up After Colonoscopy and Polypectomy.[135]

It's important to recognize the difference between TAs and SSPs. Whereas TAs have a regular, tubular gland pattern (**Figure 3.4**), SSPs have irregular serrations that look a bit like shark teeth. The significance of SSPs is that they can give rise to CRC through a different pathway than TAs. Up to 30% of sporadic CRCs arise from the so-called CpG island methylator phenotype (CIMP) via serrated polyps. CRC from this pathway is also more likely to have the "BRAF mutation," more likely to be right sided in location, and more likely to be poorly differentiated when compared to cancers that arise from TAs. For this reason, the ACG guidelines are a little more aggressive about surveillance of SSAs compared to TAs (also because there is less published data on the natural history of SSAs). As shown in **Figure 3.3**, patients with one or 2 SSPs, each <10mm in diameter should have repeat colonoscopy in 5-7 years. When that number rises to 3-4 small SSPs you need to move surveillance up to 3-5 years. At 5-10 SSPs surveillance colonoscopy should be performed at 3 years. Finally, if there are >10 SSPs then repeat colonoscopy in one year.

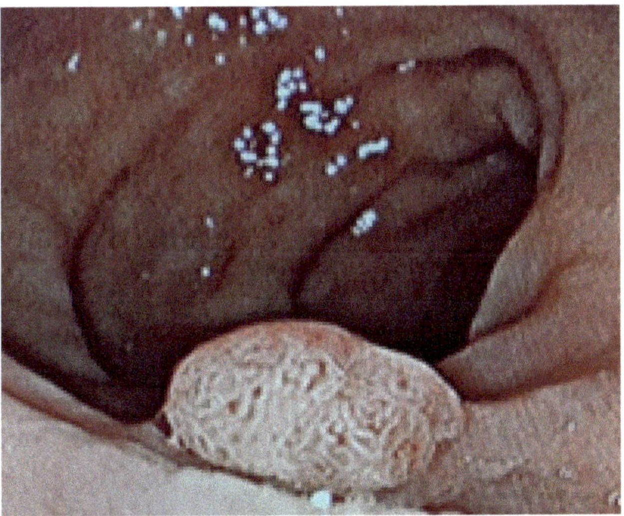

Figure 3.4 Tubular adenoma displaying characteristic tubuli in lighter areas surrounded by darker vessels in a typical tubular gland pattern.
Image source: Hetal A. Karsan, MD.

What if this had been a larger polyp removed in piecemeal fashion? In that case, he would need follow-up colonoscopy in 6 months. Same would apply for piecemeal resection of a TA. There's no messing around when there's a chance that the polyp is not fully resected. Meta-analysis reveals a 20% risk for recurrent neoplasia with piecemeal resection compared to 3% for *en bloc* removal with endoscopic mucosal resection (EMR) of large polyps.[136] Additional studies have also found an increased risk of recurrence with piecemeal removal of polyps $\geq$20 mm compared to *en bloc* resection with EMR.[137,138] Furthermore, a prospective study with over 1400 patients who underwent colonoscopy with polypectomy found that larger polyps (10-20 mm) had a significantly increased incomplete resection rate compared with small (5-9 mm) neoplastic polyps (17.3% vs 6.8%; *P*= 0.003). Moreover, almost half (47.6%) of large (10-20 mm) sessile serrated polyps were incompletely removed.[139] Wow. Thus, if a 20 mm or larger size polyp (either TA or SSP) is resected in piecemeal fashion, then a follow-up colonoscopy is needed for another look in 6 months' time. Due to the importance for resecting polyps completely, there is separate set of recommendations on this topic from the USMSTF on CRC,[140] which we review elsewhere.

What about serrated polyposis syndrome? You should suspect this condition when there are 5 or more SSPs that are proximal to the sigmoid colon with at least 2 of the polyps 10mm or larger. If there are over 20 SSPs in the colon, then that's another indicator of serrated polyposis syndrome. Note that the diagnosis of serrated polyposis syndrome is based upon the cumulative history of polyps. It's vital to obtain and review prior colonoscopies and associated pathology reports. Also, *any* number of SSP proximal to the sigmoid colon in an individual who has a first degree relative with serrated polyposis syndrome must also be suspected. In these cases, the risk of malignant transformation is high and thus mandate close surveillance, ranging from follow up at 1 to 3 years depending upon the findings of the last exam.[141]

So, what about the patient's question about lifestyle modifications. Is there anything he can do to lower his risk of for future CRC? Unfortunately, the evidence for lifestyle modifications such as altering diet, losing weight for those who are obese, smoking cessation, or exercise to reduce risk of metachronous neoplasia is lacking. There is no conclusive evidence to say that any of these changes can help reduce his future risk. Nonetheless, it is useful for patients to make these lifestyle modifications to help other aspects of their health. For now, surveillance colonoscopy has the best evidence to reduce future risk of CRC in patients with significant polyps.

Case 3.5: Bad Prep

A 48-year-old woman undergoes a direct access screening colonoscopy to the cecum. Unfortunately, she had stool debris noted throughout the colon, which was unable to be cleared despite vigorous irrigation and suctioning as shown in **Figure 3.5**. There were no polyps identified. Immediately afterwards, she was instructed to repeat the colonoscopy to be scheduled in the near future with a better bowel cleansing regimen due to the suboptimal examination. She notes that she felt very hungry while fasting and opted to eat a sandwich for dinner. She also admits to having difficulty completing the prep as instructed. She reports that she "couldn't drink that entire gallon last night" and "won't try that again."

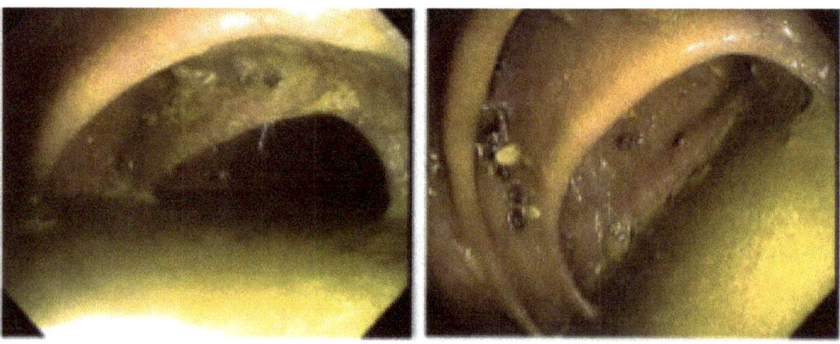

Figure 3.5. Colonic images: Descending colon (left) and ileocecal valve (right). Image source: Hetal A. Karsan, MD.

Know your guidelines!
1. Does she really need to repeat the colonoscopy?
2. What was wrong with the prep dosing as prescribed?
3. Are there other options available for prepping?
4. What is the relationship between bowel prep quality and adenoma detection rate?

Case 3.5: What do the guidelines say?

Source: U.S. Multi-Society Task Force on Colorectal Cancer 2014 Guidelines on Optimizing Adequacy of Bowel Cleansing

We've all seen poor preps. Like, *a lot* of poor preps! As an aside, GI docs are a unique breed of professionals who have no compunctions about grabbing lunch after a morning of working within pools of liquid stool. At any rate, how can you rectify this mess?

As discussed in the ACG guidelines,[142] this patient should have her colonoscopy repeated with a better bowel cleansing preparation within 1 year since she had an inadequate examination to the cecum and no polyps were identified. The ACG functionally defines an inadequate prep as one that makes it difficult to find polyps greater than 5 mm. The better part of valor would be to pull the scope out after reaching the rectosigmoid and acknowledging this is a battle that needs to be fought another day. One tip that we use is having the intake nurse "get a direct visual" if there is any doubt. That is, the check-in or intake nurse requests specific details from the patient on the most recent effluent. If there is any doubt about it, then we ask the patient to use the toilet without flushing and have the nurse take a look in the toilet. If it appears murky or muddy with some solids in there, we cancel right away. But if time permits (especially if the patient was originally scheduled in the morning), then we ask the patient to drink another bowel preparation and return in the afternoon to get the colonoscopy accomplished if at all possible (not always pragmatic, but worth considering).

There were some problems in the preparation for her colonoscopy. If instructed properly, patients are more likely to comply. A randomized, prospective trial showed that a pre-endoscopy patient education improved bowel preparations, reduced cancellations and was also cost-effective.[143] Both oral and written patient education instructions for all components of the colonoscopy are strongly recommended and certainly could have helped this patient. For example, years ago one of your authors noticed that many of his patients would stop their prep early because they thought having watery stool meant they were done. But they didn't realize the stool needs to be clear and yellow, *like pee*, not just watery. So, a picture was created to instruct patients on what do look for when taking their prep, as shown in **Figure 3.6**.[144] Variations of this original picture are all over the Internet now (just type in "bowel prep clear yellow" into Google and you'll see them).

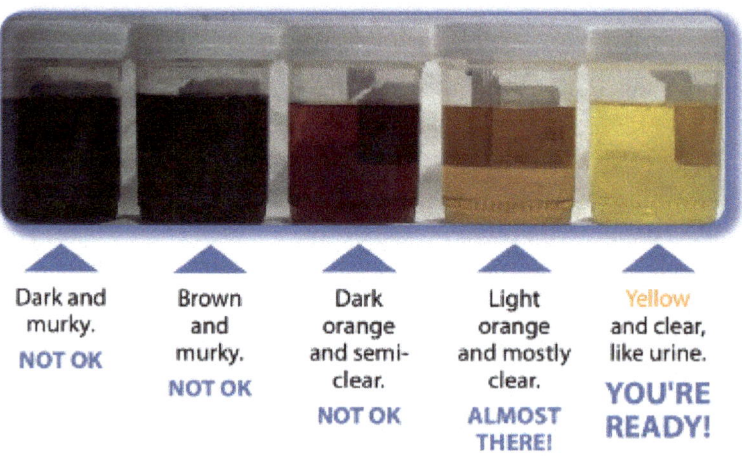

Figure 3.6. Is My Prep Working? This instruction page was developed for an educational booklet that was tested in a randomized trial and proven to improve bowel prep.[144] Patients need to understand that emitting liquid stool is not enough; the stool must be yellow and clear, like urine, to ensure an ideal prep (image developed by B. Spiegel and photographed in his kitchen way back in 2008 using food coloring!).

Back to the patient. Why did she eat that sandwich? That certainly didn't help her prepare the colon. Some advocate for a clear liquid diet the day before a colonoscopy, which is fine. However, a more liberalized diet including low-residue or full liquids can be entertained in motivated and compliant patients.

Most important is that the prep dosing should have been split over 2 days. Contrary to the persistent belief among those who trained in the single-dose prep era, split dosing over 2 days is associated with increased willingness to repeat the preparation for the future compared to the day before regimen. Moreover, split dosing is essential to clean the right side of the colon where small intestinal chyme can build up and form a thin layer, especially when the entire prep is taken the night before the procedure. Thus, flat lesions can get overlooked with a single-dose evening prep. This issue can be simply explained to patients: if you aren't clean, then you're setting yourself up to have polyps missed. "Let's make this one and done," we like to say. "Let's do this right, and do it once."

Time is of the essence for split dose preps. This first dose can be consumed earlier in the day to allow better sleep. But timing the second dose is most critical. It's been shown that prep quality varies inversely with duration of the interval between the last dose of prep and the start of the colonoscopy. The longer the time interval, the less chance of cleaning the right colon.[2] Not surprisingly, studies have revealed that split dosing, where the second dose of the split preparation begins 4-6 hours before the colonoscopy increases ADR significantly.[145,146]

The ACG guidelines also provide a strong recommendation for same-day bowel prep regimen, where the entire prep is given the morning of an afternoon colonoscopy. In fact, a prospective study showed that a same-day regimen provided more effective mucosal cleansing with less sleep disturbance, better tolerance and was preferred by patients compared with split dosing.[147]

In addition, there are several low-volume bowel cleansing preparations available, which tend to be better tolerated and associated with increased willingness to undergo future colonoscopies. It is important to keep in mind that these low-volume preps require adequate supplementation with 2 to 3 liters of clear liquids to prevent dehydration. Selecting the best regimen should be tailored to the patient's history and medications (e.g., history of chronic constipation or narcotic use which can lead to suboptimal preps) and adequacy from prior colonoscopies. Some patients will just need a little more to clear out effectively. Although patients often complain about the discomfort and inconvenience of bowel preps, it's important to recognize that the efficacy of bowel preparation is vital to ensure a complete exam and lower overall cancer risk.

By the way, it is important to document the adequacy of the bowel preparation on each examination after all efforts have been made to clear any residual debris. With modern scopes that have improved irrigation and suctioning, at least 85% of colonoscopies should have adequate bowel cleansing to identify polyps greater than 5 mm, which are typically more significant than smaller polyps. This means that the colonoscopist will not have the patient come back earlier than screening or surveillance guidelines dictate.

With these items in mind, this patient had a repeat colonoscopy (**Figure 3.7**) and was spick and span!

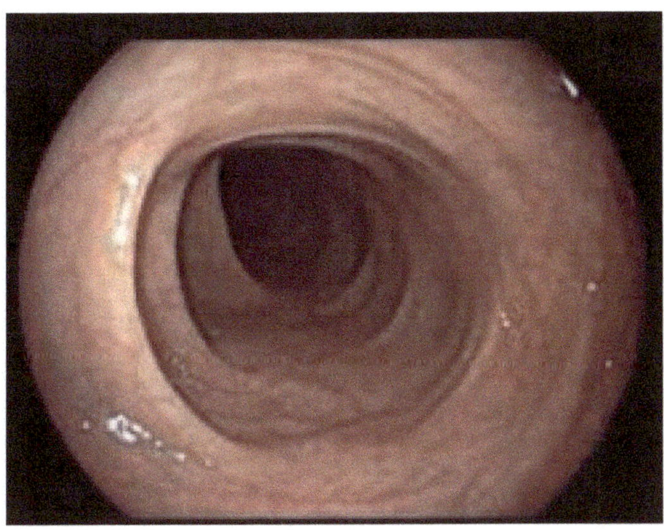

Figure 3.7. Image from repeat colonoscopy. Image source: Hetal A. Karsan, MD

Case 3.6: A Big Polyp

A 54-year-old woman presents to you for first-time CRC screening. There is no family history of CRC or other cancers. You perform colonoscopy and discover the ~3.5 cm lesion, below, in the ascending colon. No other lesions are identified.

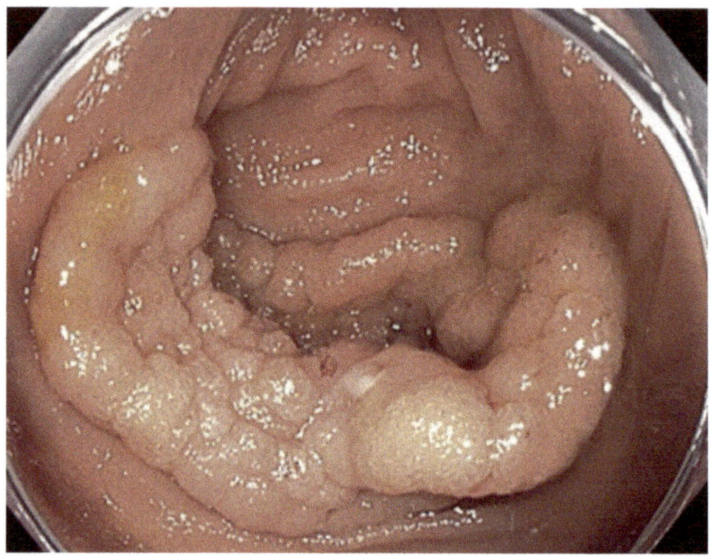

Figure 3.8. Large polyp in ascending colon. Image source: ACG guidelines.[139]

Know your guidelines!

1. How would you describe this lesion?
2. What are you going to do about it?

Case 3.6: What do the guidelines say?

Sources: ACG 2020 Endoscopic Removal of Colorectal Lesions Guidelines; ACG 2020 Endoscopic Recognition and Management Strategies for Malignant Colorectal Polyps Guidelines; ACG 2015 Quality Indicators for Colonoscopy Guidelines

Although polypectomy is an everyday occurrence for gastroenterologists, it's easy to forget how amazing it is that removing polyps can prevent cancer and save lives. Seriously. With one simple maneuver we can massively change people's lives for the better. That's big time!

So, how much does polypectomy help? The National Polyp Study, which dates back to 1993, found that endoscopic removal of adenomas lowers CRC mortality by 50% compared to controls not receiving polypectomy.[148] Moreover, CRC incidence has dropped over the past decade in part due to enhanced CRC screening and timely polypectomy of premalignant tumors.[149]

Polypectomy lowers CRC mortality by 50%

It's worth asking why colonoscopy doesn't provide 100% risk protection. There are several explanations. First, if you don't see a polyp then you won't be able to remove it. This speaks to the importance of ensuring excellent bowel preparation (as discussed in the last vignette), achieving cecal intubation, *slowly* pulling back during the procedure (ideally, for at least a 6-minute withdrawal time),[150] and looking very carefully for all polyps. Of course, adhering to these best practices will not completely eliminate CRC risk, but the more quality indicators achieved, the lower the risk of future cancer.[151] The ACG recommends that cecal intubation be achieved in $\geq$95% of cases, and that bowel prep be considered adequate in $\geq$85% of cases, where "adequate" means you can easily visualize a $\geq$5mm polyp.[146] Anything short of these markers should be addressed with local quality improvement initiatives. In addition, the ACG emphasizes that the overall adenoma detection rate (ADR) should be $\geq$25% for an individual endoscopist, with $\geq$20% for female and

$\geq$30% for male patient populations.[122] You should anticipate that these goal rates will increase in the future as more data continues to trickle in.

That said, it's also vital to ensure complete and safe technical removal of colorectal polyps and that will be the focus of this discussion. The ACG guidelines on endoscopic polypectomy offer a comprehensive review.[137] Here, we will address only a part of that expansive and authoritative document. Like all the other ACG guidelines, be sure to check out the original source for all the details.

First off, when you encounter a polyp during colonoscopy, start by examining its size, shape, and surface morphology. Be sure to photo-document and describe these features in your report, especially for lesions $\geq$1cm. The ACG guidelines recommend applying the Paris classification system because it can help risk stratify lesions for cancer risk.[139] According to this system, there are 2 overarching types of polyps: Type 0, or superficial lesions; and Types 1-5, the advanced cancers. The details are beyond what we'll cover here, but **Figure 3.9** breaks down the Type 0 lesions, ranging from pedunculated, to sessile, minimally elevated, flat, minimally depressed, and ulcerated lesions. Note that over 40% of small, depressed lesions contain submucosal invasive cancer and pretty much all large (>2cm) depressed lesions are cancerous.[152] That's why it's so important to determine if there is evidence of depression and document that in your note.

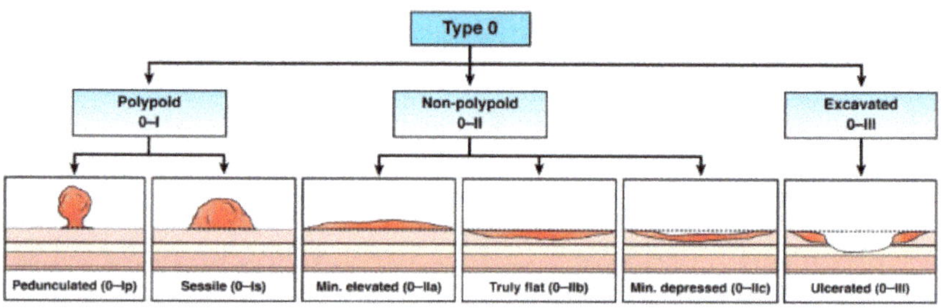

Figure 3.9 Subtypes of Type 0 Lesions According to Paris Classification.

When a lesion falls in the "non-polypoid" spectrum and is >1cm in diameter it's called a "laterally spreading tumor" (LST). When an LST has a nodular surface, it's called a "granular type" LST, as seen in the current vignette. In contrast, smooth-surfaced LSTs are termed "non-granular." **Figure 3.10** shows examples. Making this distinction is important because granular LSTs have a *lower* risk of harboring submucosal invasion (5.9%) vs non-granular, smooth-surfaced LSTs (11.7%).[153] The lesion in the current vignette looks more granular given its multiple nodules and lobes, which actually portends a better prognosis than if the lesion had been completely smooth. We'll get back to managing this vignette soon.

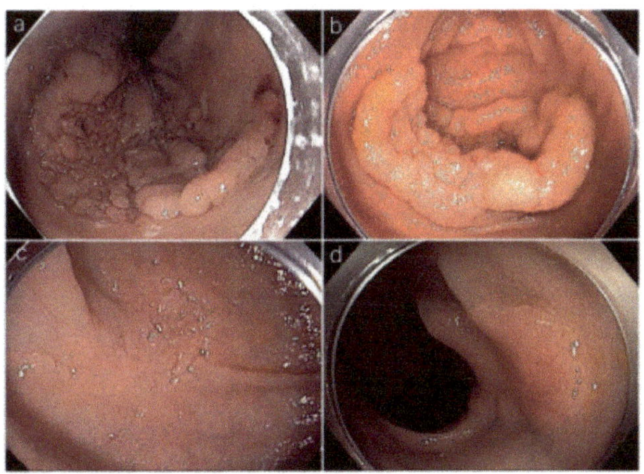

Figure 3.10 Examples of laterally spreading tumors (LSTs). Panels (a) and (b) demonstrate examples of granular LSTs, whereas panels (c) and (d) show non-granular (i.e., smooth-surfaced) LSTs. It's the smooth, non-granular lesions that have a higher risk of harboring underling cancer.

There are other surface features to consider when attempting to divine the type of polyp and underlying cancer risk. For example, a large polyp that is flat, has indistinct borders, a "clouded surface," and/or a mucous cap might indicate a sessile serrated lesion. A lesion that does not lift easily with fluid injection may be a sign of deep submucosal invasion.

Narrow band imaging (NBI) can also help to assess other important surface features of colonic lesions. The NBI International Colorectal Endoscopic (NICE) classification system was designed to classify polyps as serrated vs conventional based on surface features.[154] Furthermore, the system involves careful assessment of the pit pattern which is known to correlate with certain types of lesions.[155] **Figure 3.11** shows common pit patterns as described in the NICE classification. These are best viewed with use of dye spray (i.e., chromoendoscopy), although that is uncommonly used in clinical practice.

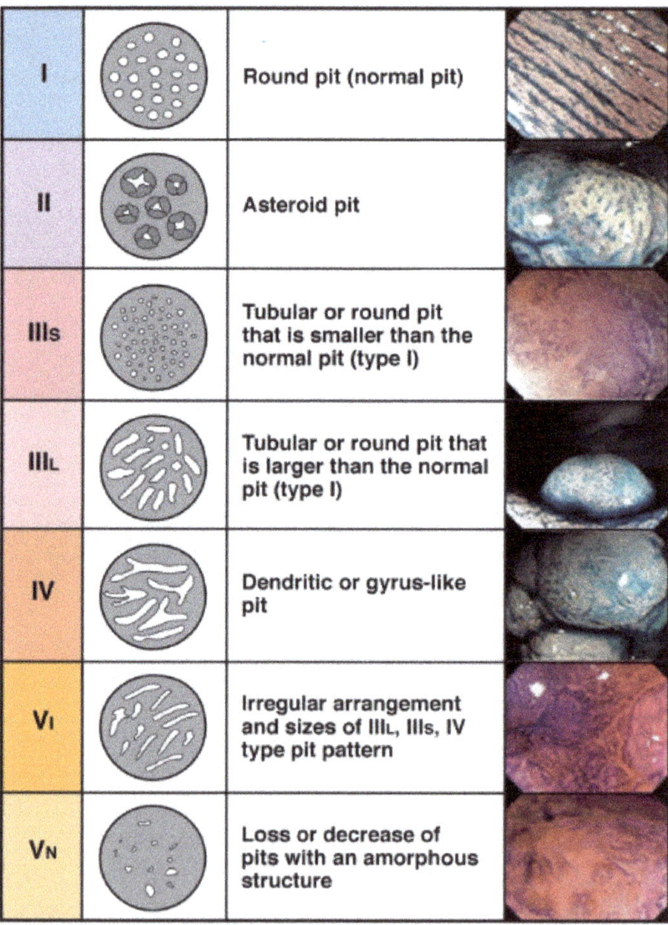

Figure 3.11 NICE classification of polyp pit patterns.

Starting at the top, type I pits are regular, round pits that are normal in appearance. From there, things begin to change. Type II pits are fantastically described as "asteroid" pits that look stellar in nature. These can also be normal, or may occur with serrated, hyperplastic, or inflammatory polyps. But normally, type II pits do not indicate dysplasia or malignant changes. In contrast, type III-V pits suggest dysplasia or malignancy. The type III pits are tubular and (surprise) suggest a tubular adenoma. Type IV pits are dendritic or "gyrus-like" and suggest a tubulovillous or villous adenoma. Type V lesions feature an irregular assortment of pits and/or loss of pits altogether with an amorphous structure. These are highly concerning for cancer. As an aside, it won't be long until artificial intelligence (AI) systems can quickly and accurately distinguish the pit patterns without relying upon the human eye. Stay tuned for that to become more primetime.

Let's take a step back and evaluate the decision tree for managing superficial colorectal lesions. The ACG guidelines offer a comprehensive algorithm which is shown in **Figure 3.12.**

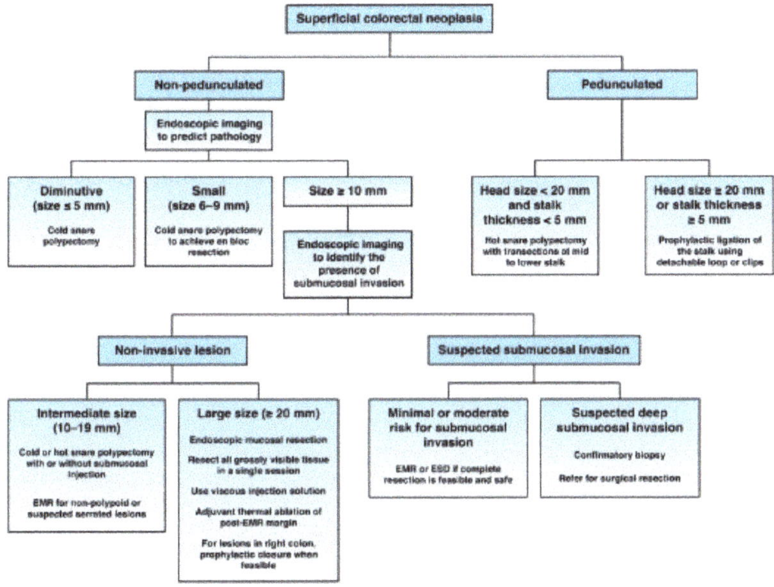

Figure 3.12 ACG Algorithm for Managing Colorectal Lesions.[139]

It all starts with distinguishing pedunculated from non-pedunculated lesions. If the lesion is pedunculated, then the management depends on the size of the head and stalk. If the head size is less than 2 cm and the stalk less than 5 mm, then hot snare polypectomy (i.e., with electrocautery) is recommended. Larger polyps have a higher risk of post-polypectomy bleeding and therefore should undergo prophylactic ligation with a detachable loop or clip prior to excising the tumor to reduce bleeding risk.

Non-pedunculated lesions take up a lot more space on the decision tree. Start by examining the surface features to help determine risk of submucosal invasion. Next, consider the size of the lesion. This is where things have changed a lot in the past 2 decades. It used to be that we'd pull out biopsy forceps for most small lesions and only grab the snare for polyps that were on the larger size. Moreover, we'd usually apply a hot snare to lesions which, we were taught, lowered the risk of bleeding. That's all changed. Now, any lesion less than 1cm should be removed with cold snare polypectomy, ideally with a 0.3mm wire rather than the larger 0.47 mm wire. This approach minimizes damage to the mucosa, is safe, and optimizes *en bloc* resection rather than piecemeal resection from picking away with biopsy forceps. Also, in the past, some endoscopists would use hot forceps to excise polyps. That's a no-go now. Just avoid hot forceps because it damages the tissue and leads to incomplete resections when compared to cold snare. The guidelines concede that for very small lesions, such as those <2 mm, you can consider using "jumbo" cold forceps if snare polypectomy is technically infeasible. Basically, cold forceps are okay for very small polyps if you can get the entire lesion in one bite. Otherwise, you should be using a cold snare to obtain adequate margins whenever possible.

If the non-pedunculated lesion is ≥1cm in diameter, then next stratify based on whether there are concerning surface features, such as those already discussed. In the current vignette, the lesion is non-pedunculated, larger than 1cm in diameter, and nodular in appearance, consistent with a granular LST that does not show obvious surface evidence of submucosal invasion.

If there is no sign of submucosal invasion, then the algorithm distinguishes lesions that are 10-19 mm from those greater than or equal to 20 mm in diameter. That is, for those lesions less than 20 mm, a cold snare polypectomy with or without submucosal injection or endoscopic mucosal resection (EMR), particularly if you suspect a sessile serrated lesion with indistinct borders.

If the lesion is ≥2cm in diameter, then EMR with a viscous injection solution or endoscopic submucosal dissection (ESD) are recommended, typically in partnership with a colleague who is experienced in advanced polypectomy (maybe that's you, in which case, just do it yourself!). You should also apply adjuvant thermal ablation of the post EMR margin with either argon plasma coagulation (APC) or by using the electrocauterized snare tip to zap the surrounding area of a large resection. However, bear in mind that this ablative technique should *not* be applied to visible adenomatous tissue which should instead be removed with cold snare, not buzzed directly. For lesions in the right colon

that are large, consider prophylactic closure with clips if feasible, and certainly if there is any concern of perforation following resection. For example, if you see a "target sign," which appears like a white circular rim of muscularis propria at the resection site, it means you went too deep and there's an increased risk of perforation. In that case, lay down some clips.[156] For a lot more information on the technical details of EMR and ESR, refer to the full guidelines.

If you do an EMR for a ≥2 cm lesion (as in this case), then be sure to follow-up with a surveillance colonoscopy in 6 months to inspect the area and clean up any residual adenomatous tissue that might emerge. If the site looks good, then repeat again in 1 year, and then

After EMR follow-up at 6 months, 1-year, and 3-years (assuming no recurrence)

in 3 years. If there is residual tissue, then perform surveillance every 6-12 months until there is no evidence of recurrence at the site. Then go back to the 1-year and 3-year interval schedule.

If you have serious concerns of submucosal invasion based on surface inspection, then snare polypectomy ain't enough. You need to either send the patient for EMR or ESD for endoscopic resection if there is minimal or moderate risk, or straight to surgical resection if there is high risk for submucosal invasion.

Finally, what are the risk factors for post-polypectomy bleeding, and what do the guidelines recommend for lowering the risk of bleeding? Because we can never pass up a good mnemonic (or even a bad mnemonic ;-), we offer "POO RED" as one way to remember the various risk factors of post-polypectomy bleeding, shown in **Figure 3.13**.

P endunculated lesions
O ne centimeter diameter (or greater)
O ral anticoagulants

R ight-sided lesions
E lderly with comorbidities (esp. cardiovascular or renal)
D eep or spreading lesions

Figure 3.13 Risk Factors for Post-Polypectomy Bleeding Spell Out "POO RED."

In the absence of these risk factors, it is not cost-effective to apply routine prophylactic treatments to polypectomy sites. However, for large lesions, particularly those exceeding 2 centimeters in the proximal colon, randomized trial data indicate that prophylactic clipping reduces the risk of delayed bleeding from 7.2% to 3.7%

when compared to no clipping.[157] In contrast, prophylactic coagulation of visible vessels after EMR has not been shown to lower post-polypectomy bleeding.[158]

Case 3.7: Family History of Cancer

A 45-year-old woman presents to your clinic with concerns about her personal cancer risk due to a family history of various cancers. She reports that her mother was diagnosed with CRC at the age of 52 and her younger brother was diagnosed with CRC at the age of 40. Additionally, her maternal aunt was diagnosed with endometrial cancer in her late 50s. Given this significant family history, the patient is worried that she may be at increased risk for developing cancer. She is otherwise asymptomatic, has an unremarkable physical exam, and no evidence of anemia on blood tests.

Know your guidelines!

1. What diagnosis are you most concerned about?
2. What are the next steps for managing this patient?

Case 3.7: What do the guidelines say?

Source: U.S. Multi-Society Task Force 2014 Guidelines on Lynch Syndrome; ACG 2015 Guidelines on Genetic Testing and Management of Hereditary GI Cancer Syndromes

What percentage of cancers are related to a hereditary syndrome? Think on that for a moment because it's an important number to have tucked away in your mind. We scope a lot, see lots of polyps, occasionally find cancers…but we don't always remember to look for underlying hereditary syndromes. It's vital to diagnose these syndromes not only for the sake of your patients, but also for their families. Okay, so what percentage of cancers are attributable to a hereditary syndrome? Around 5%-10%.[159] That's a lot.

Because hereditary syndromes are always lurking beneath the surface, it's important to ask your patients about a family history of cancer. Inquire about an early age at onset of polyps or cancer in all first- and second-degree relatives. Although asking about third-degree relatives may be important for a geneticist, the ACG guidelines recognize that's a bit extreme for everyday practice. But at least be sure to ask and document information about first- and second-degree relatives.

The patient in this vignette presents with a strong history of cancer in both first- and second-degree relatives. There is early-onset CRC in both her mother and brother, and her maternal aunt had endometrial cancer in her 50s. This is worrisome for a hereditary cancer syndrome, namely Lynch Syndrome (LS), an autosomal-dominant condition marked by a germline mutation in a DNA mismatch repair (MMR) genes that boosts personal and familial risk of cancer, including CRC and endometrial cancer as seen here.

You should suspect LS using the 3-2-1-1 rule based on the Amsterdam II criteria: at least **3** relatives must have an LS-related cancer, spanning at least **2** successive generations, with **1** cancer occurring in first-degree relative and at least **1** occurring before age of 50.[136] This patient meets those criteria.

Patients with LS are at high risk for developing many types of cancer (**Table 3.4**). This occurs due to microsatellite instability (MSI) resulting from defective MMR genes and a subsequent loss of the MMR proteins MLH1, MSH2, MSH6, and/or PMS2. For a patient like this one, it's important to consider genetic testing to evaluate for possible LS, typically in partnership with a genetic counselor. Start by testing the MMR genes for evidence of pathogenic variants or mutations. In addition, if the index tumors are available from affected family members, then direct immunohistochemical (IHC) testing can be performed on the tumor itself. This involves examining tumor tissue for MSI or loss of expression of MMR proteins using IHC analysis.

Table 3.4. *Cancers Associated with Lynch Syndrome*

Colorectal cancer
Endometrial cancer
Ovarian cancer
Gastric cancer
Ureteral, renal pelvis, and bladder cancer
Small intestinal cancer
Biliary tract cancer
Pancreatic cancer

Patients at risk for LS should be screened by colonoscopy at least every 2 years beginning at ages 20-25 years. Those found to have a confirmed mutation should undergo annual colonoscopy. Note that LS-related CRC tends to occur at a much earlier age (as early as 40-45 years old) compared to sporadic CRC (~65-70 years) and also tends to be more right-sided in origin. The lifetime risk of CRC in LS is around 22% to 74% across trials, with higher rates in those with MSH6 mutations compared to those with MLH1 and MHS2, which portend a somewhat lower (yet still elevated) risk.[136] If there is evidence of CRC or recurrent premalignant polyps despite multiple polypectomies, then colectomy with ileorectal anastomosis is warranted in lieu of partial colectomy. You don't want to leave anything behind given the very high risk of progression to CRC.

It's important to work with a multidisciplinary team when managing LS. For example, hysterectomy and bilateral salpingo-oophorectomy should be offered to women who are known LS mutation carriers and who have finished childbearing, optimally at age 40-44 years of age. Screening for endometrial cancer and ovarian cancer should also be offered starting at age 30-35 years. From a GI standpoint, be sure to perform endoscopy with gastric biopsies starting at age 30-35 and every 3-5 years thereafter if there's a family history of gastric or duodenal cancer. Test and treat for *H. pylori* whenever you perform biopsies in these patients. **Table 3.5** summarizes the surveillance guidelines for LS.

Table 3.5 *Screening Guidelines for LS. Table obtained from ACG / US Multi-Society Task Force Guidelines on Genetic Evaluation and Management of Lynch Syndrome.*[160]

Intervention	Recommendation	Strength of Recommendation
Colonoscopy	Every 1-2 y beginning at age 20-25 y or 2-5 y younger than youngest age at diagnosis of CRC in family if diagnosis before age 25 y. Considerations: Start at age 30 y in MSH6 and 35 in PMS2 families Annual colonoscopy in MMR mutation carriers	Strong recommendation: Level of evidence: well-designed and conducted cohort or case-controlled studies from more than 1 group with cancer. GRADE rating: moderate
Pelvic examination with endometrial sampling	Annually beginning at age 30-35 y	Offer to patient: Level of evidence: expert consensus GRADE rating: low
Transvaginal ultrasound	Annually beginning at age 30-35 y	Offer to patient: Level of evidence: expert consensus GRADE rating: low
EGD with biopsy of the gastric antrum	Beginning at age 30-35 y and subsequent surveillance every 2-3 y can be considered based on patient risk factors	Offer to patient: Level of evidence (V): expert consensus GRADE rating: low
Urinalysis	Annually beginning at age 30-35 y	Consideration: Level of evidence (V): expert consensus GRADE rating: low

Case 3.8: Fundic Gland Polyposis

A 42-year-old man presents for recurrent and severe dyspepsia and nausea for the past several months. He describes the upper abdominal discomfort as a gnawing sensation that worsens after meals. He has noticed an increase in bloating, belching, and occasional heartburn. Over-the-counter antacids, proton pump inhibitors, and *H. pylori* eradication have not resolved his symptoms. On exam there is mild tenderness in the epigastrium but no palpable masses or organomegaly. There are no signs or symptoms of anemia and complete blood count is normal. However, due to the persistence of symptoms, he undergoes an upper endoscopy for further evaluation which reveals the findings in **Figure 3.14,** along with an ampullary adenoma.

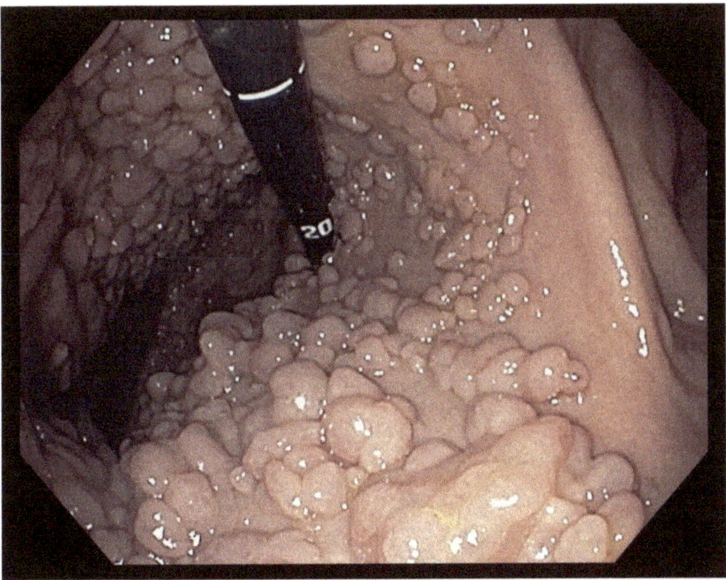

Figure 3.14 Findings on Upper Endoscopy. Image source: Phil Fleshner, MD and Kavya Reddy, MD.

Know your guidelines!

1. What diagnosis are you most concerned about?
2. What test is warranted now?

Case 3.8: What do the guidelines say?

Source: ACG 2015 Guidelines on Genetic Testing and Management of Hereditary GI Cancer Syndromes

This patient needs a colonoscopy right away. If you were to do that test, then you might see this the image in **Figure 3.15**, below.

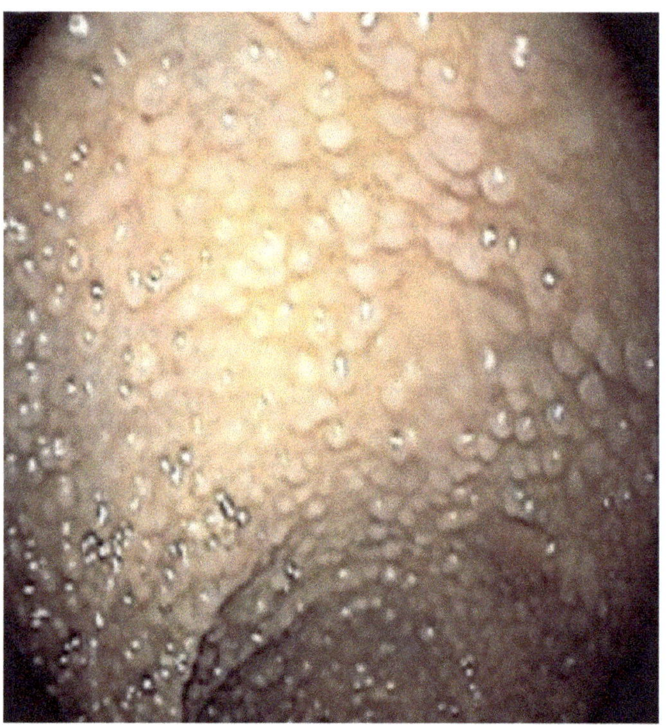

Figure 3.15 Carpet of Polyps.[172]

You've probably known since med school that when you see a carpet of polyps in the colon, like the image above, the diagnosis is probably familial adenomatous polyposis (FAP). That much is easy enough. But what causes FAP? How do we distinguish FAP from attenuated FAP (AFAP)? What's the difference between FAP and MUTYH-associated polyposis (MAP)? What's the association between FAP and fundic gland polyps? And what are the next steps in management? Thank goodness the ACG guidelines have us covered!

212

FAP is an autosomal-dominant syndrome resulting from a mutation in the APC tumor suppressor gene that presents with ≥ 100 colorectal adenomas, increased risk of CRC, foregut adenomas, and risk of several extraintestinal malignancies. You just know FAP when you see it; no need to hand count all the polyps in that picture. On the other hand, you might see a *lot* of polyps, but not the 100+ carpeting the entire visualized colon. When you see ~25+ adenomas, but something short of the full carpet of adenomas, then think about AFAP which arises from a mutation of the APC gene that isn't quite as severe as full-blown FAP.

In contrast to FAP and AFAP, MAP is an autosomal recessive disorder marked by ≥ 25 colorectal adenomas. MAP results from biallelic MUTYH mutations, where MUTYH is a base excision repair gene involved in cleaning up oxidative damage to DNA.

But this patient clearly has FAP based on the colonoscopy. To confirm, send him to a genetic counselor to discuss FAP and undergo testing for APC gene mutations. Patients like this require annual colonoscopy or flexible sigmoidoscopy beginning at puberty. In contrast, patients with AFAP or MAP require a full colonoscopy every year since the lesions in those conditions can be more sporadic and possibly right sided in comparison to FAP, where a flex sig is adequate.

CRC is inevitable in FAP if the colon remains intact, with a mean onset at age 39 years. By the time an FAP patient reaches 45 years old, there is nearly a 90% risk of having CRC. However, survival is greatly improved when patients undergo close monitoring and timely colectomy. The ACG guidelines indicate that surgery is immediately indicated if there is evidence of cancer, and non-urgently indicated when there are multiple adenomas that are >6 mm, a significant rise in adenoma number over serial colonoscopies, any adenoma found to have high-grade dysplasia, or inability to adequately survey the colon due to multiple diminutive polyps covering the surface.

As with Lynch Syndrome, patients with FAP are at risk for extracolonic malignancies and need to be monitored carefully throughout their lives. Screening for gastric and proximal small bowel tumors should be performed with upper endoscopy started at age 25-30 years. Subsequent surveillance intervals vary between 6 months and 4 years depending on the stage of duodenal polyposis using detailed criteria we won't discuss here (see the guidelines if you're curious). Gastric biopsies are important to monitor for evidence of mucosal dysplasia or other premalignant lesions, and careful inspection of the duodenum and ampulla are vital. In fact, the most common cause of death after CRC is duodenal or ampullary cancer. Also, keep an eye out for fundic gland polyposis of the stomach, as occurred in this case. Earlier in the book we discussed how fundic gland polyps are no big deal when associated with PPI therapy. But beware when fundic gland polyps occur in the setting of FAP because they can progress to cancer. This patient was on PPIs, but don't expect PPIs to cause 30+ fundic gland polyps and an ampullary adenoma. That needs to trigger suspicion for underlying FAP.

There are a bunch of other cancers that can form with FAP, including papillary thyroid cancer, adrenal adenomas, small bowel cancers, osteomas, nasopharyngeal cancer, congenital hypertrophy of the retinal pigmented epithelium, and epidermoid cysts of the skin. Those are great to know for board exams but also emphasize the importance of working with a multidisciplinary team when managing FAP. **Figure 3.16** offers a way to memorize the FAP-related cancers. It spells out CAPSTONE, which has nothing really to do with FAP. If you don't like that, then you can also try

"ADENOMA," which gets most of the cancers but misses thyroid.
So, pick whichever you like!

C ongenital hyperplasia of retinal pigment
A drenal adenoma
P apillary thyroid cancer
S mall bowel cancer
T hyroid cancer (again!)
O steoma
N asopharyngeal cancer
E pidermoid cyst of the skin

OR...

A drenal adenoma
D uodenal (small bowel)
E pidermoid cyst
N asopharyngeal
O steoma
M edullablastoma
A mpullary adenoma

Figure 3.16 The FAP-related cancers spell out CAPSTONE or ADENOMA.

Case 3.9: Surveillance after CRC Resection

A 68-year-old man develops new onset constipation with bloating over the past few weeks. He also was found to have iron deficiency anemia and is referred to you for a colonoscopy by his primary care physician. He mentions that prior to this episode he had always felt well. Therefore, he did not previously get a colonoscopy as requested by his primary care provider. On today's colonoscopy he is noted to have the descending colon lesion pictured in **Figure 3.17** with inability to safely pass the colonoscope proximally. After the procedure, you inform the patient that the lesion is concerning for CRC and will require timely surgical resection given the impending obstruction.

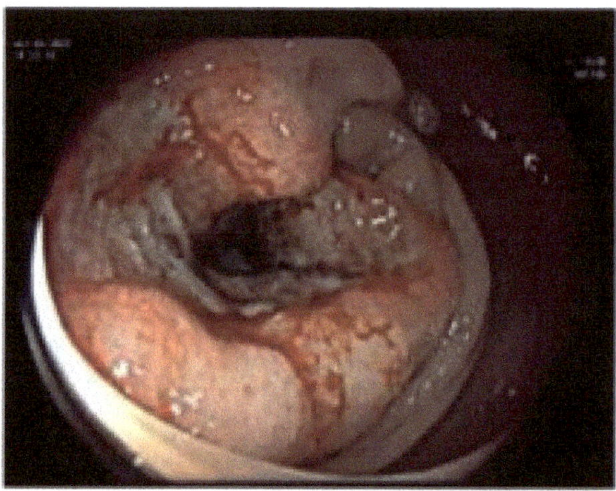

Figure 3.17 Descending colon lesion. Image source: Hetal A. Karsan, MD.

Know your guidelines!

1. What else should be done prior to surgical resection?
2. How often should he receive future surveillance colonoscopies after surgical resection?

Case 3.9: What do the guidelines say?

Source: Colonoscopy Surveillance After Colorectal Cancer Resection: Recommendations of the US Multi-Society Task Force on Colorectal Cancer.

Before we delve into postoperative CRC surveillance guidelines,[161] it is important to review best practices for pre-operative evaluations. Optimally, the entire colon should be examined before surgery to remove any polyps and look for any other tumors. However, in this case the scope was unable to be safely passed through the obstructing lesion. If available, this patient could have received a preoperative computed tomography colonography (CTC) to exclude synchronous neoplasms proximal to the obstructed region.[162] It may be particularly useful to obtain a CTC with intravenous contrast to evaluate for distant metastases, while at the same time looking for other proximal synchronous lesions. Of course, you want to remind your radiology colleagues not to overinflate those patients with an obstructing lesion due to the risk of perforation. Although CTC is the more sensitive and preferred option, a double-contrast barium enema may suffice under these circumstances depending upon local availability.[163]

> A preop CTC synchronous neoplasms proximal to an obstructing colon cancer

As an aside, you may recall that the USMSTF endorsed CTC as a second-tier option for those unwilling or unable to undergo colonoscopy or FIT.[164] Let's say an average risk person gets a CTC, which is negative. Assuming this person wants to continue with this route of CRC screening, when should the next screening CTC be performed? A gut reaction (yep, another pun intended) might be to do it again in 10 years; however, a screening CTC should be performed every 5 years if negative.

> CTC screening is performed every 5 years, not every 10 years

However, CTC is not available everywhere, so it would be reasonable to just ensure the patient proceeds with a post-operative colonoscopy 3 to 6 months after resection, which is noted in the guideline. Moreover, even if the patient gets a preop CTC showing no other significant tumors, then he should still get a high-quality colonoscopy within 3 to 6 months postoperatively to clear the road and remove any polyps that the initial scope did not get to see. How about after that? It has been shown that more intensive follow up improves overall survival.[165] Thus, it is not surprising that patients who have had CRC resection tend to get colonoscopies more often than recommended.[166] This patient should receive another high-quality colonoscopy 1 year after his clearing colonoscopy. If that is negative, then repeat another one in 3 years (i.e., 4 years after surgery or perioperative colonoscopy) and then in 5 years (i.e., 9 years after surgery or perioperative colonoscopy). After that it should be done every 5 years depending on the overall health of the patient. Of course, if polyps are found and removed, then future colonoscopy surveillance intervals are guided by the general polyp surveillance guidelines (peel back some pages in this book and review it again for a refresher).

Rectal cancer behaves a little differently than the typical colon cancer because it's more prone to localized recurrence, which in turn can be decreased by total mesorectal excision and neoadjuvant therapy (chemoradiation).[167] Although total mesorectal excision is typically performed, sometimes this radical surgery may not be conducted due to concerns of increased mortality and morbidity, especially decreased quality of life. Thus, patients with localized rectal cancer who have undergone transanal excision or transanal endoscopic microsurgery should be followed more closely with EUS (or sigmoidoscopy depending upon local availability) every 3-6 months for the first 2-3 years after surgery, since they are higher risk for localized recurrence than those who have received total mesorectal excision. Note that this localized surveillance strategy for rectal cancer is an adjunct to the recommended colonoscopic surveillance for metachronous neoplasia described above.

Thus, it is very important that you remind patients that they will need to be rescoped somewhat regularly after surgical resection. Interestingly, postoperative colonoscopy is associated with improved overall survival but not necessarily cancer-related mortality. The differences in all-cause mortality versus colon cancer-specific specific mortality can be explained by the fact that providers select healthier patients to get colonoscopy surveillance. So, these generally healthier colon cancer survivors tend to be watched more closely in general regarding their overall health and non-oncologic medical care and in turn, live longer.[168]

Case 3.10: Gastric Subepithelial Lesion

A 63-year-old man presents to his primary care physician with dyspepsia. He is tested for *H. pylori* which is negative, and is then treated with PPI therapy for 8 weeks without much benefit. He is now sent to you by his PCP for endoscopy. You decide to scope. There is no erosive esophagitis or ulceration found, but you discover the lesion in the antrum of the stomach, shown below in **Figure 3.18**. The lesion measures roughly 1.5 cm in diameter.

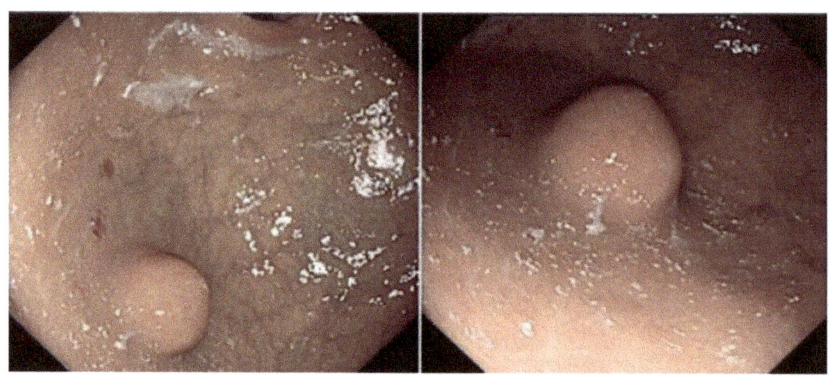

Figure 3.18 Lesion in Antrum of Stomach. Image source: Simon Lo, MD.

Know your guidelines!

1. What is this lesion most likely to be?
2. What is the next step in evaluating this lesion?

Case 3.10: What do the guidelines say?

Source: ACG 2023 GI Subepithelial Lesion Guideline

As endoscopists, we frequently discover subepithelial lesions (SELs) throughout the GI tract. The stomach is a common source of SELs, as seen in the current vignette, so it's important to know the full range of gastric SELs and their management. Fortunately, the ACG has us covered with its 2022 SEL guideline.[169] We'll go through the decision tree in a moment, but first, a picture quiz.

Take a look at the **Figure 3.19**. It's a ~1cm lesion encountered in the antrum of the stomach. What's the diagnosis?

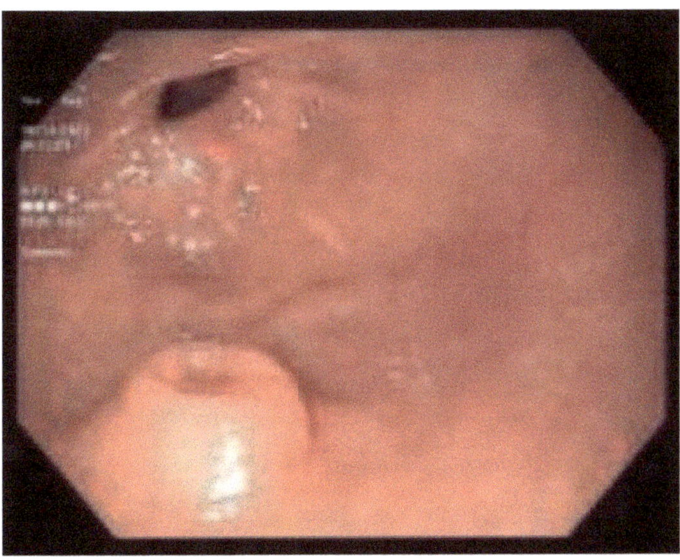

Figure 3.19 Lesion in Antrum of the Stomach. Image source: Hetal A. Karsan, MD

You probably know this one. But if not, let's knock it out quick. There is a central umbilication on this lesion which reveals the diagnosis: it's a pancreatic rest, or heterotopic pancreatic tissue buried in the wall of the antrum. The central umbilication is like a proto pancreatic duct. This finding is harmless and should be left alone.

Okay, let's go back now to the picture in the vignette. Here it is again:

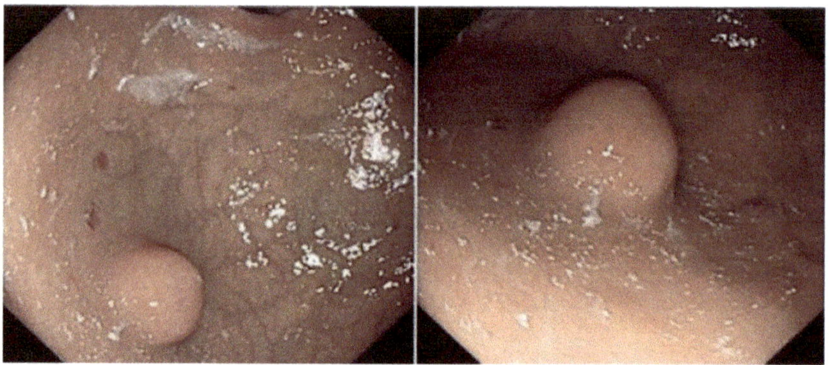

Without knowing anything else, what's the most likely diagnosis for this lesion? Back when we were fellows the answer might have been a leiomyoma. In those dark ages, we didn't recognize the difference between leiomyomata and gastrointestinal stromal tumors (GISTs), but now we can distinguish them with immunohistochemical testing of endoscopic ultrasound (EUS)-obtained biopsy specimens (more on that soon).

It turns out that the most common SEL in the stomach is a GIST, not a leiomyoma. Oh, by the way, we sometimes hear people talk about "GIST tumors." The "T" in GIST stands for tumor, so it's already contained in the word GIST. Sorry, just a pet peeve of ours. While we're at it, don't say "dysplastic adenoma." All adenomas are dysplastic. Or say "malignant melanoma," because all melanomas are... well, you get the gist!

When should you be worried about a GIST? There are a few features that increase the risk of malignancy and they're listed in **Table 3.6**.

Table 3.6 *Features of GIST That Increase Risk of Malignancy.*

Heterogenous echotexture
Size >3cm
Size increasing on serial images
Irregular margins
Evidence of cystic-appearing spaces within the lesion
Echogenic foci within the lesion
Malignant appearing lymph nodes in region

When 2 or more of these features are present, then the sensitivity for malignancy is 80% or higher. In contrast, absence of any suspicious EUS findings means cancer risk is much lower, ranging from 0% to 11%.[170]

To make sense of the ACG SEL guidelines, it's important to first review the layers of the GI tract with a focus on endosonographic correlates of these anatomic layers. Check out **Figure 3.20**, for a depiction of the EUS layers of the GI tract. Anatomically, there is only one epithelial layer in the GI tract. But endosonographically, this structure is divided into 2 layers: the superficial and deep mucosa. The superficial mucosal layer is hyperechoic (or white) on EUS, and results from the sound waves bouncing off the mucosa interface. Next, the hypoechoic (or dark) second layer represents the deep mucosa which contains the muscularis mucosa, which should not be confused with the soon-to-come fourth layer, or the muscularis propria. Recall that the muscularis mucosa is a very thin layer of muscle that does not support motility, but instead squeezes the glands of the GI tract to help jettison their contents into the lumen. The hyperechoic third layer is the submucosa. The thick hypoechoic fourth layer is the muscular propria, which produces motility through contraction of its inner circular and outer longitudinal segments. Finally, the fifth hyperechoic layer is the serosa or adventitia (latter in the case of the esophagus), depending on where you are in the GI tract. You'll recall that the esophagus does not have a serosa whereas the rest of the GI tract does.

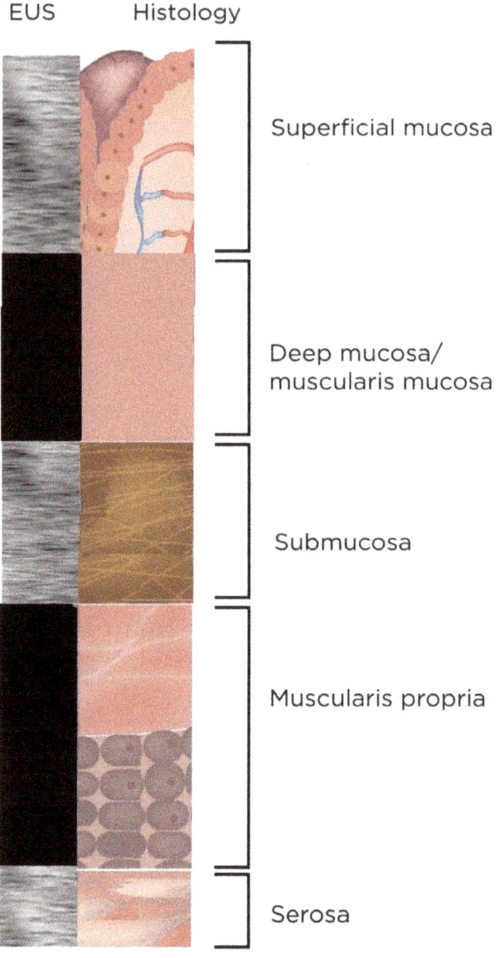

Figure 3.20 EUS Layers of the Stomach.

So, as we mentioned, this lesion is probably a GIST and is most likely arising from the fourth layer of the stomach. In contrast to leiomyomata, which originate from smooth muscle cells and stain positive for actin on immunohistochemistry, GISTs arise from the interstitial cells of Cajal and stain positive for

CD117, or c-kit, which is a tyrosine kinase receptor. This receptor can be targeted by imatinib mesylate which is the treatment of choice for non-operable GISTs. We'll come back to the management of GIST (and other SELs) in a little bit. But first, let's walk through the ACG algorithm for SELs, starting with the first part of the decision tree shown in **Figure 3.21.**

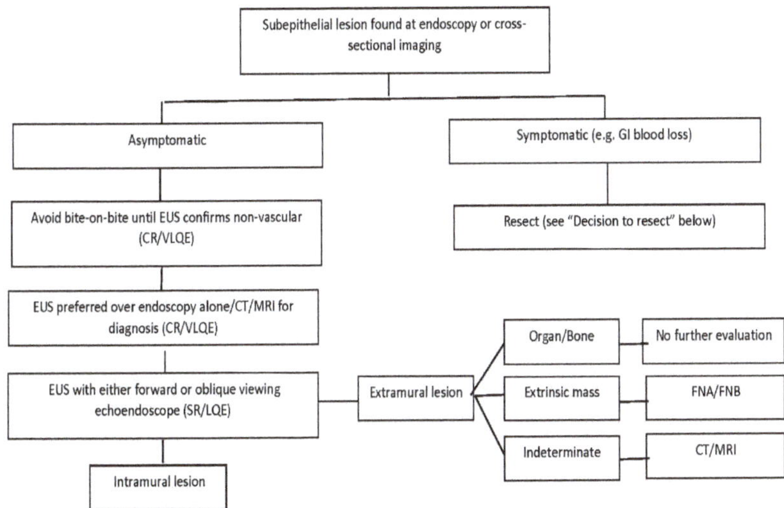

Figure 3.21 Part I of ACG SEL Algorithm (We've broken this massive algorithm into parts, because, well, it's a monster).

The algorithm starts simply enough: you encounter an SEL on endoscopy and/or cross-sectional imaging. What next? First, determine whether it's bleeding or not. If the SEL has broken through the mucosa and is bleeding out, then definitive therapy is required for both diagnosis and treatment. These lesions should be resected either surgically or endoscopically. We'll skip those details until later.

If the SEL is not bleeding, then EUS is warranted to confirm the presence of an intramural vs extramural lesion and to determine whether there are vascular components. This approach is preferred

225

over mucosal biopsies, which are unlikely to be diagnostic since, by definition, the lesion is subepithelial. Some people try the "bite-on-bite" technique where they take one mucosal biopsy, then biopsy again within the footprint of the previous biopsy as if to burrow into the lesion one bite after another. That just doesn't cut it (so to speak...). Better to perform EUS and properly evaluate the lesion's origin and characteristics. For example, if you're looking at a vascular lesion, like a gastric varix, then you obviously shouldn't dig in with forceps. Or, if it's an extramural lesion, like a compressing organ or an extrinsic mass, then the biopsy has no chance of reaching the source anyway. Extrinsic lesions account for roughly one-third of SELs. So, holster your forceps at this stage and pull out the EUS (or ask someone who knows EUS to help you out), which brings us to part II of the ACG algorithm shown in **Figure 3.22**.

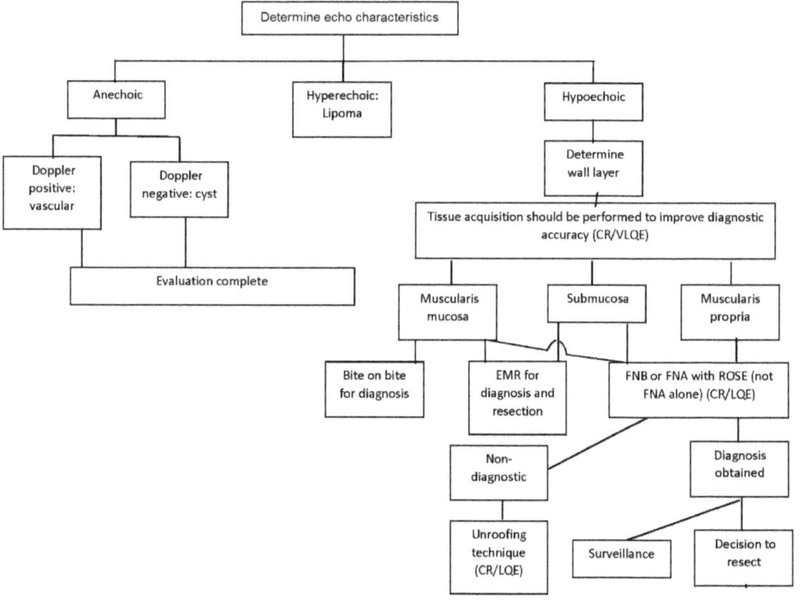

Figure 3.22 Part II of ACG SEL Algorithm.

Next determine whether the EUS reveals an anechoic, hyperechoic, or hypoechoic SEL. If it's anechoic, then you're either dealing with a vascular lesion or a cyst; Doppler evaluation can distinguish

the two. If it's hyperechoic, then you've got a lipoma arising from
the third endosonographic layer. If it's hypoechoic, then determine its layer of origin and perform
tissue acquisition to diagnose the lesion. A lesion
arising from the muscularis mucosa (layer 2) can be
reached with regular biopsy forceps using the bite-on-bite technique (the only time this approach works), whereas a submucosal
(layer 3) or muscular propria (layer 4) lesion requires fine needle
biopsy (FNB) with rapid on-site evaluation (ROSE) or fine needle aspiration (FNA). These biopsies will either be diagnostic, in
which case a decision must be made on whether to
resect, or nondiagnostic, in which case the guidelines suggest trying again by "unroofing" the mucosa with jumbo biopsy forceps to get a better sample.

There is an exception to this guideline. If you find a soft, "pillowy,"
and mobile SEL that easily indents under pressure from the biopsy
forceps, then you're probably dealing with a lipoma.
If this lesion is also yellowish then it's a presumptive lipoma and EUS is not required. In contrast,
a yellowish lesion that is firm and does not exhibit
a "pillow sign" cannot be diagnosed as a lipoma on
endoscopy alone. Bear in mind that granular cell tumors and certain neuroendocrine tumors (NETs) like carcinoids
can also exhibit a yellow appearance.

At some point, you'll need to decide whether the SEL should be
resected. We've already talked about the need to remove bleeding
lesions and the lack of need to resect lipomas or pancreatic rests. If
the lesion is a GIST, a NET, or in the esophagus and/or GEJ,
then part III of the ACG algorithm provides guidance, as
shown in **Figure 3.23**.

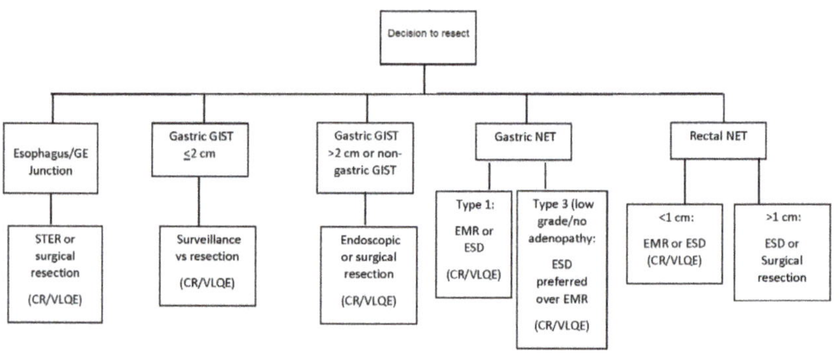

Figure 3.23 Part III of ACG SEL Algorithm.

The decision to resect an SEL depends on its location, tissue type, and size. If an SEL is found in the esophagus or GEJ, then it should be removed with either submucosal tunneling endoscopic resection (STER) or surgical resection. SELs in this location are typically either a leiomyoma or GIST. Since the esophagus is a small-caliber organ, a growing SEL is likely to cause symptoms and should be managed proactively both for diagnostic and therapeutic purposes.

If the SEL is in the stomach and is found to be a GIST, then next determine its size. Lesions >2cm should be resected either endoscopically or surgically depending on local expertise and preference. If the gastric GIST is ≤2cm, then the guidelines recommend surveillance vs resection; there is insufficient evidence to definitively recommend one approach over the other. The decision of whether to resect or monitor depends on presence of the concerning features discussed earlier (see **Table 3.5**). For example, a gastric GIST that is only 1cm in diameter might still have cystic spaces, echogenic foci, or irregular borders, and should therefore be considered for resection even if falls below the 2cm threshold for definitive resection. Finally, if the GIST is non-gastric then it should be resected no matter the size.

If the SEL is a gastric NET, such as a carcinoid tumor, then it's important to distinguish whether it is a Type 1, Type 2, or Type 3 NET. It would be easier if there were just one type of gastric NET but, alas, there are 3. So, what's the difference? Type 1 occurs in the setting of chronic atrophic gastritis with hypergastrinemia. These lesions have a relatively lower risk of malignant transformation compared to other types of gastric NETs. Type 2 NETs occur in the setting of multiple endocrine neoplasia-1 (MEN-1) syndrome or Zollinger Ellison Syndrome; they also have a relatively low rate of malignant transformation and often occur in bunches, making them less feasible to resect. Type 3 NETs are sporadic, unrelated to hypergastrinemia, and carry a much higher risk of malignant transformation (up to 50% 5-year mortality) compared to Types 1-2.[171] The guidelines recommend performing either endoscopic mucosal resection (EMR) or endoscopic submucosal dissection (ESD) for lesions Type 1 NETs and prefer ESD for Type 3 NETs.

Finally, rectal NETs should also be resected and the exact management depends on size. For smaller rectal NETs, defined as <1cm, the guidelines recommend either EMR or ESD, whereas larger NETs should undergo either ESD or surgical resection.

And that does it for Volume I of G2G. Congrats on making it to the end. Now, take the lumps and bumps quiz and then we'll see you in Volume II!

Lumps and Bumps Quiz

1. Which of the following is true about fecal immunochemical testing for colon cancer?

    a) FIT detects peroxidase activity in stool
    b) Unlike guaiac-based tests, FIT is approved by the USPSTF
    c) FIT is less specific for CRC than DNA based stool tests
    d) The positive predictive value of FIT for colon cancer is roughly 20%
    e) FIT should be repeated every other year in patients at average risk for CRC

2. Which of the following is true about multitarget stool DNA (mt-sDNA) testing for colon cancer?

    a) Only 4% of patients with a positive mts-sDNA test will be found to have CRC
    b) If a patient has a positive mt-sDNA test followed by a normal colonoscopy, then repeat colonoscopy is warranted in 3 years
    c) In addition to suspecting colon cancer, a positive mt-sDNA test should also increase suspicion for a foregut aerodigestive cancer
    d) Current FDA-cleared mt-sDNA testing does not include a FIT component
    e) The sensitivity of one-time mt-sDNA testing for colon cancer exceeds 95%

3. At what age should you stop routine screening for colorectal cancer?

    a) 75 years
    b) 76 years
    c) 85 years
    d) 86 years
    e) 90 years

4. A 38-year-old man presents for colon cancer screening. His father was diagnosed with colon cancer at age 53. When should this patient obtain his first screening colonoscopy?

    a) Now
    b) When 40 years old
    c) When 43 years old
    d) When 45 years old
    e) When 50 years old

5. For the patient in the question above, how often should surveillance colonoscopy be performed if the index procedure is normal?

    a) Annually
    b) Every 3 years
    c) Every 5 years
    d) Every 7 years
    e) Every 10 years

6. Which of the following is not an example of an advanced polyp?

    a) 10mm tubular adenoma
    b) 5mm villous adenoma
    c) 5mm tubular adenoma with high-grade dysplasia
    d) 8mm sessile serrated lesion
    e) 5mm sessile serrated lesion with dysplasia

7. Which of the following does the ACG consider to be a marker for a high-quality colonoscopy?

    a) Bowel preparation is adequate to identify any polyps >5mm in diameter
    b) Performed by an endoscopist with an adenoma detection rate of at least 35%
    c) Performed by an endoscopist with a cecal intubation rate of at least 90%
    d) Withdrawal time of at least 8 minutes

8. A patient at average risk for colon cancer is found to have 2 tubular adenomas on screening colonoscopy that are completely resected, each measuring <10mm. When should surveillance colonoscopy be performed next?

a) 1 year
b) 3 years
c) 5 years
d) 7 years

9. A patient at average risk for colon cancer is found to have 3 tubular adenomas on screening colonoscopy with sizes 3mm, 5mm, and 10mm. When should surveillance colonoscopy be performed next?

a) 1 year
b) 3 years
c) 5 years
d) 7 years
e) 10 years

10. A patient at average risk for colon cancer is found to have an 8mm adenoma with high-grade dysplasia on screening colonoscopy that is completely resected. When should surveillance colonoscopy be performed next?

a) 6 months
b) 1 year
c) 3 years
d) 5 years

11. A patient at average risk for colon cancer is found to have a 20mm tubular adenoma on screening colonoscopy that is incompletely resected. When should surveillance colonoscopy be performed next?

a) 6 months
b) 1 year
c) 3 years

d) 5 years

12. A patient at average risk for colon cancer is found to have 12 hyperplastic polyps in the sigmoid colon and rectum that are completely resected, each <10mm. When should surveillance colonoscopy be performed next?

   a) 6 months
   b) 1 year
   c) 3 years
   d) 5 years
   e) 10 years

13. A patient at average risk for colon cancer is found to have a 12mm hyperplastic polyp in the sigmoid colon that is completely resected. When should surveillance colonoscopy be performed next?

   a) 1 year
   b) 3-5 years
   c) 5-10 years
   d) 7-10 years
   e) 10 years

14. Approximately what percentage of sporadic colon cancers arise from serrated polyps?

   a) 1%
   b) 5%
   c) 15%
   d) 30%
   e) 50%

15. Compared to colon cancers that arise from tubular adenomas, which of the following is true about cancers that arise from serrated polyps?

a) They arise from the CpG island methylator phenotype
b) They are more likely to be left-sided in location
c) They are less likely to be poorly differentiated
d) They are less likely to feature a BRAF mutation

16. In which of the following scenarios should you suspect serrated polyposis (SSP) syndrome?

a) 4 sessile SSPs proximal to the sigmoid colon, each <10mm
b) 12 SSPs scattered throughout the colon, 1 of which is >10mm
c) 3 SSPs in the proximal colon that are each >10mm
d) 8 SSPs in the left colon, of which 2 are >10mm
e) 1 SSP in the right colon that is 5mm in a patient with a first degree relative with confirmed serrated polyposis syndrome

17. Which of the following lifestyle modifications has been definitively shown to lower risk of colorectal cancer?

a) Smoking cessation
b) Weight loss for those who are obese
c) Exercise
d) Avoiding alcohol
e) None of the above

18. Patients prepping for colonoscopy should be told that their stool should end up looking more like:

a) Pee
b) Poo

19. Compared to single-dose evening preps, split dose preps:

a) Are less well tolerated
b) Are associated with higher adenoma detection
c) Are especially better at cleaning the left colon
d) Require a lower cumulative volume of ingested liquid

20. Which of the following bowel preparations is most effective for a late afternoon colonoscopy?

a) Single dose the night before the procedure

b) Single full dose the morning of the procedure
c) Split dose beginning the evening before the procedure
d) Split dose beginning the morning of the procedure

21. According to the National Polyp Study, what is the risk reduction for colon cancer afforded by polypectomy?

a) 10%
b) 30%
c) 50%
d) 70%

22. A patient is found to have a 10mm depressed, non-polypoid lesion in the right colon. What is the approximate pre-test probability the lesion harbors submucosal invasive cancer?

a) 5%
b) 10%
c) 20%
d) 30%
e) 40%

23. A 10mm flat but non-depressed lesion is found in the right colon. It has indistinct borders, a "clouded surface," and an overlying mucous cap. Which of the following lesions is most likely?

a) Tubular adenoma
b) Tubulovillous adenoma
c) Sessile serrated lesion
d) Carcinoid tumor
e) Adenocarcinoma

24. Which of the following polyp pit patterns is most concerning for cancer risk?

a) Wide and round pits
b) Dendritic pits

c) Tubular pits
d) Asteroid pits

25. Which of the following polyps should be removed with a "hot" electrocautery snare?

    a) 15mm pedunculated polyp
    b) 15mm non-pedunculated polyp
    c) 10mm non-pedunculated polyp
    d) 7mm non-pedunculated polyp
    e) Diminutive (<5mm) polyp

26. Colonoscopy reveals a 20mm non-pedunculated polyp with a granular surface without ulceration. Which of the following is the most appropriate next step?

    a) Cold snare polypectomy without submucosal injection
    b) Submucosal injection followed by cold forcep piecemeal polypectomy
    c) Hot forcep piecemeal polypectomy
    d) Endoscopic mucosal resection
    e) Refer directly for surgical resection

27. You remove a large polyp in the right colon using snare polypectomy with submucosal injection but notice a small amount of residual adenomatous-appearing tissue at the edge of the polypectomy site. Which of the following is the most appropriate technique to remove the marginal tissue?

    a) Remove with hot forceps
    b) Ablate with argon plasma coagulation
    c) Ablate with electrocauterized snare tip
    d) Remove with cold snare

28. A single, 25mm, laterally spreading tumor in the right colon is removed with endoscopic mucosal resection. When should you next perform surveillance colonoscopy?

    a) 3 months
    b) 6 months
    c) 12 months

d) 3 years
e) 5 years

29. Which of the following is not a risk factor for post-polypectomy bleeding?

    a) Use of oral anticoagulants
    b) Left-sided lesion
    c) Cardiovascular comorbidities
    d) Pedunculated lesion
    e) Lesion >1cm in diameter

30. Which of the following is not a component of the Amsterdam II criteria for Lynch syndrome (LS)?

    a) At least 3 first- or second-degree relatives have an LS-related cancer
    b) LS-related cancers found in at least 2 successive generations
    c) At least one family member has an LS-related cancer occurring before age 40
    d) At least 1 LS-related cancer in a first-degree relative

31. Which of the following colorectal cancer screening strategies is recommended for patients with Lynch Syndrome?

    a) Flexible sigmoidoscopy annually starting at puberty
    b) Colonoscopy every 1-2 years starting at age 20-25
    c) Colonoscopy every 3-4 years starting at age 30-35
    d) Colonoscopy annually starting at age 30-35

32. In addition to screening for CRC in patients with Lynch Syndrome, which of the following is also a guideline recommend screening strategy?

    a) Ultrasound of the thyroid every 3 years, starting at age 40
    b) Chest x-ray every 2 years, starting at age 40
    c) Pelvic examination with endometrial sampling annually, starting at age 30-35
    d) Upper endoscopy every 1-2 years, starting at age 35-40

33. Which of the following forms of hereditary polyposis is inherited in an autosomal recessive pattern?

   a) Lynch Syndrome
   b) Familial Adenomatous Polyposis (FAP) Syndrome
   c) Attenuated FAP Syndrome
   d) MUTYH-Associated Polyposis (MAP) Syndrome

34. Which of the following colorectal cancer screening strategies is recommended for patients with FAP?

   a) Flexible sigmoidoscopy annually starting at puberty
   b) Colonoscopy every 1-2 years starting at age 20-25
   c) Colonoscopy every 3-4 years starting at age 30-35
   d) Colonoscopy annually starting at age 30-35

35. Which of the following extraintestinal lesions is associated with FAP?

   a) Congenital hyperplasia of retinal pigment
   b) Medullary thyroid cancer
   c) Prostate cancer
   d) Breast cancer
   e) Uterine cancer

36. After CRC, which of the following is the next most common cause of cancer-related mortality in patients with FAP?

   a) Small bowel cancer
   b) Adrenal cancer
   c) Papillary thyroid cancer
   d) Nasopharyngeal cancer

37. A patient at average risk for colorectal cancer undergoes computerized tomographic colonoscopy (CTC). When should the next CTC be performed?

   a) 1 year
   b) 3 years
   c) 5 years
   d) 7 years
   e) 10 years

38. A patient presents with a large bowel obstruction and is found to have an obstructing cancer in his sigmoid bowel. He is brought to surgery and undergoes left hemicolectomy. When should a follow-up "clearing" colonoscopy be performed?

   a) Within 1 month
   b) Within 2 months
   c) Within 3-6 months
   d) Within 12 months

39. A patient receives a postoperative "clearing" colonoscopy after surgery for a malignant large bowel obstruction. It does not show any other colonic lesions and demonstrates an intact anastomosis. When should the next surveillance colonoscopy be performed?

   a) 6 months
   b) 1 year
   c) 2 years
   d) 3 years

40. A patient is found to have rectal cancer which is removed with transanal excision. Which of the following is the recommended postoperative surveillance strategy?

   a) Colonoscopy in 3-6 months
   b) Colonoscopy in 12 months
   c) Endoscopic ultrasound in 3-6 months
   d) Endoscopic ultrasound in 12 months

41. Upper endoscopy reveals a subepithelial antral lesion with a central umbilication. What is the most likely diagnosis?

a) Gastrointestinal stromal tumor
b) Schwannoma
c) Leiomyoma
d) Pancreatic rest
e) Lipoma

42. Which of the following is the most common subepithelial lesion of the stomach?

a) Gastrointestinal stromal tumor
b) Schwannoma
c) Leiomyoma
d) Pancreatic rest

43. Which of the following is a high-risk feature of a GIST?

a) Size > 1cm
b) Homogenous echotexture
c) Anechoic spaces within the lesion
d) Smooth margins

44. Which of the following histological layers corresponds with the second endosonographic layer?

a) Muscularis propria
b) Mucosa interface
c) Deep mucosa
d) Submucosa
e) Serosa

45. A 2cm subepithelial lesion is found in the upper stomach on endoscopy. Endoscopic ultrasound reveals an anechoic mass. Which of the following is the most likely diagnosis?

a) Gastric varix
b) Lipoma
c) GIST
d) Pancreatic rest
e) Glomus tumor

46. A 2cm subepithelial lesion is found in the upper stomach on endoscopy. Endoscopic ultrasound reveals a hyperechoic mass. Which of the following is the most likely diagnosis?

a) Gastric varix
b) Lipoma
c) GIST
d) Pancreatic rest
e) Leiomyoma

47. Beyond what size should a gastric GIST be resected?

a) 1cm
b) 2cm
c) 3cm
d) 4cm
e) 5cm

48. A patient with longstanding pernicious anemia and hypergastrinemia is found to have multiple, small, subepithelial gastric lesions. Which of the following is the most likely diagnosis?

a) Type I neuroendocrine tumors (NET)
b) Type II NETs
c) Type III NETs

49. Which of the following gastric NETs has the highest risk of malignant transformation?

a) Type I NET
b) Type II NET
c) Type III NET

50. Beyond what size should a rectal GIST be resected?

a) 1cm
b) 2cm
c) 3cm
d) 4cm
e) 5cm

Lumps and Bumps Quiz Answers

1.	B	18.	A	35.	A
2.	A	19.	B	36.	A
3.	D	20.	B	37.	C
4.	B	21.	C	38.	C
5.	C	22.	E	39.	B
6.	D	23.	C	40.	C
7.	A	24.	B	41.	D
8.	D	25.	A	42.	A
9.	B	26.	D	43.	C
10.	C	27.	D	44.	C
11.	A	28.	B	45.	A
12.	E	29.	B	46.	B
13.	B	30.	C	47.	B
14.	D	31.	B	48.	A
15.	A	32.	C	49.	C
16.	E	33.	D	50.	A
17.	E	34.	A		

Acknowledgments

We thank the authors of the ACG guidelines covered in this book who provided expert review on their sections: Michael Camilleri, MD, MACG; William D. Chey, MD, FACG; Evan S. Dellon, MD, MPH, FACG; Samir Gupta, MD; Brian C. Jacobson, MD, MPH, FACG; David A. Johnson, MD, MACG; Charles J. Kahi, MD, MSc, FACG; Philip O. Katz, MD, MACG; Brian E. Lacy, MD, PhD, FACG; Paul Moayyedi, MB ChB, PhD, MPH, FACG; Mark Pimentel, MD, FACG; Nicholas J. Shaheen, MD, MPH, MACG; Aasma Shaukat, MD, MPH, FACG; Michael F. Vaezi, MD, PhD, MSc(Epi), FACG; and Arnold Wald, MD, MACG. We also wish to thank the following people who provided original images used in this book: Jonathan Gotfired, MD; Simon Lo, MD, FACG; Kavya Reddy, MD; Ali Rezaie, MD, MSc; and Philip Fleshner, MD. In addition, we thank the ACG Board of Trustees and Practice Parameters Committee for their continued work on developing guidelines and supporting the GI community. Lastly, we thank the ACG editorial team for their production and editing work on this book: Claire Neumann, Neen LeMaster, and Morgan Huntt.

Personal Dedications

H.K.: To my precious wife, Lina, my beloved children, Sonia and Rajan, and my supportive parents, Arvind and Urmila, for all of their everlasting encouragement and inspiration. Nothing is possible without them. *Iamque opus exegi.* Om Shanti Shanti Shanti.

B.S.: To my wife and children for just being amazing.

MEET THE AUTHORS

Brennan Spiegel, MD, MSHS, FACG

Dr. Spiegel is the Dorothy and George Gourrich Chair in Digital Health Ethics at Cedars-Sinai, Founding Director of the Cedars-Sinai Master's Program in Health Delivery Science, and an ACG Governor for Southern California. He is the immediate past Editor-in-Chief for *The American Journal of Gastroenterology* and inaugural Editor-in-Chief for the *Journal of Medical Extended Reality*. Dr. Spiegel has published widely in the fields of health services research, digital health, use of virtual reality in medicine, and clinical gastroenterology across a range of topics. Together with Dr. Karsan, he also wrote the "Acing the GI Board Exam" series of books.

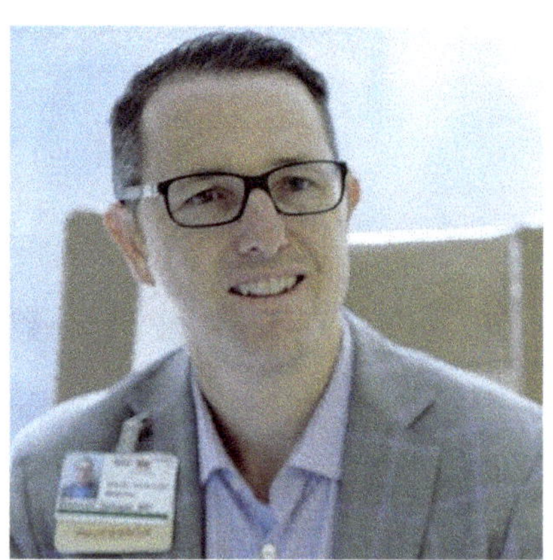

Hetal A. Karsan, MD, FACG

Dr. Karsan is the Chair of Medical Education for United Digestive and Adjunct Professor of Medicine in the Division of Digestive Diseases at Emory University. He serves as the Chair of the Credentials Committee, International Governor, and Governor of Georgia for the ACG. He is the immediate past Editor of the Red Section and Associate Editor for *The American Journal of Gastroenterology*. He has practiced for more than twenty years in both private and academic settings, while actively maintaining board certifications in Gastroenterology, Transplant Hepatology and Internal Medicine. Collaborating with Dr. Spiegel, he wrote the "Acing the GI Board Exam" series of textbooks.

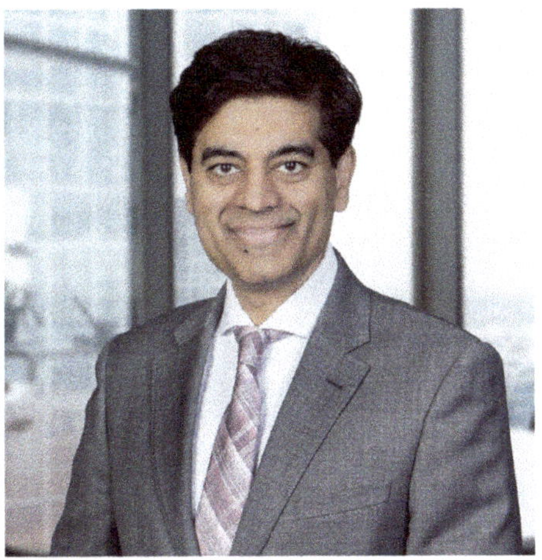

References

1. Lacy BE, Mearin F, Chang L, Chey WD, Lembo AJ, Simren M. Bowel disorders. *Gastroenterology*. 2016;150:1393-1407

2. Shah A, Talley NJ, Jones M, Kendall BJ et al. Small intestinal bacterial overgrowth in irritable bowel syndrome: A systematic review and meta-analysis of case-control studies. *Am J Gastroenterol*. 2020;115:190-201

3. Pimentel M, Saad RJ, Long MD, Rao SS. ACG clinical guideline: Small intestinal bacterial overgrowth. *Am J Gastroenterol*. 2020;115:165-178

4. Rezaie A, Buresi M, Lembo A, Lin H, et al. Hydrogen and Methane-Based Breath Testing in Gastrointestinal Disorders: The North American Consensus. *Am J Gastroenterol* 2017;112:775-784

5. Tuck CJ, Yaoa CK, Phipott HL, Brett JS. Questioning the utility of breath testing in clinical practice; *Am J Gastroenterol*. 2017;112:1886

6. Yu D, Cheeseman F, Vanner S. Combined oro-caecal scintigraphy and lactulose hydrogen breath testing demonstrate that breath testing detects oro-caecal transit, not small intestinal bacterial overgrowth in patients with IBS. *Gut*. 2011;60:334-340

7. Low K, Hwang L, Hua J et al. A combination of rifaximin and neomycin is most effective in treating irritable bowel syndrome patients with methane on lactulose breath test. *J Clin Gastroenterol* 2010;44:547–550

8. Lacy BE, Pimentel M, Brenner DM, Chey WD, Keefer LA, Long MD, Moshiree B. ACG clinical guideline: Management of irritable bowel syndrome. *Am J Gastroenterol*. 2021;116-44

9. Fodor AA, Pimentel M, Chey WD, et al. Rifaximin is associated with modest, transient decreases in multiple taxa in the gut microbiota of patients with diarrhoea-predominant irritable bowel syndrome. *Gut Microbes* 2019;10:22–33.

10. Rao SSC, Rehman A, Yu S, et al. Brain fogginess, gas and bloating: A link between SIBO, probiotics and metabolic acidosis. *Clin Transl Gastroenterol* 2018;9:162.

11. Spiegel BM, Farid M, Esrailian E, et al. Is irritable bowel syndrome a diagnosis of exclusion?: A survey of primary care providers, gastroenterologists, and IBS experts. *Am J Gastroenterol* 2010;105:848–58

12. Cash BD, Rubenstein JH, Young PE, et al. The prevalence of celiac disease among patients with nonconstipated irritable bowel syndrome is similar to controls. Gastroenterology 2011;141:1187–93.

13. Irvine AJ, Chey WD, Ford AC. Screening for celiac disease in irritable bowel syndrome: An updated systematic review and meta-analysis. *Am J Gastroenterol* 2017;112:65–76

14. Spiegel BM, DeRosa VP, Gralnek IM, et al. Testing for celiac sprue in irritable bowel syndrome with predominant diarrhea: A cost-effectiveness analysis. *Gastroenterology* 2004;126:1721–32.

15. Cash BD, Schoenfeld P, Chey WD. The utility of diagnostic tests in irritable bowel syndrome patients: A systematic review. *Am J Gastroenterol* 2002;97:2812–9.

16. Canavan C, Card T, West J. The incidence of other gastroenterological disease following diagnosis of irritable bowel syndrome in the UK: A cohort study. PLoS One 2014;9:e106478.

17. Porter CK, Cash BD, Pimentel M, et al. Risk of inflammatory bowel disease following a diagnosis of irritable bowel syndrome. *BMC Gastroenterol* 2012;12:3–10.

18. Van Rheenen PF, Van de Vijver E, Fidler V. Faecal calprotectin for screening of patients with suspected inflammatory bowel disease: Diagnostic meta-analysis. *BMJ* 2010;341:c3369.

19. Sidhu R, Wilson P, Wright A, et al. Faecal lactoferrin: A novel test to differentiate between the irritable and inflamed bowel? *Aliment Pharmacol Ther* 2010;31:1365–70.

20. Menees SB, Powel C, Kurlander J, et al. A meta-analysis of the utility of C-reactive protein, erythrocyte sedimentation rate, fecal calprotectin, and fecal lactoferrin to exclude inflammatory bowel disease in adults with IBS. *Am J Gastroenterol* 2015;110:444–54.

21. Ishihara S, Yashima K, Kushiyama Y, et al. Prevalence of organic colonic lesions in patients meeting Rome III criteria for diagnosis of IBS; a prospective multicenter study utilizing colonoscopy. *J Gastroenterol* 2012;47:1084–90.

22. Spiegel BMR, Gralnek IM, Bolus R, Chang L, Dulai GS, Naliboff B, Mayer EA. Is a negative colonoscopy associated with reassurance or improved health-related quality of life in irritable bowel syndrome? *Gastrointest Endosc* 2005;62:892-9

23.   Klem F, Wadhwa A, Prokop LJ, et al. Prevalence, risk factors, and outcomes of irritable bowel syndrome after infectious enteritis: A systematic review and meta-analysis. *Gastroenterology* 2017;152:1042–54.

24.   Havevik K, Dizdar V, Langeland N, et al. Development of functional gastrointestinal disorders after Giardia lamblia infection. *BMC Gastroenterol* 2009;9:27.

25.   Thabane M, Kottachchi DT, Marshall JK. Systematic review and meta-analysis: The incidence and prognosis of post-infectious irritable bowel syndrome. *Aliment Pharmacol The.* 2007;26:535.

26.   Dionne J, Ford AC, Yuan Y, et al. A systematic review and meta-analysis evaluating the efficacy of a gluten free diet and a low FODMAP diet in treating symptoms of IBS. *Am J Gastroenterol* 2018;113:1290–300.

27.   Moayyedi P, Quigley EM, Lacy BE, et al. The effect of fiber supplementation on irritable bowel syndrome: A systematic review and meta-analysis. *Am J Gastroenterol* 2014;109:1367–74.

28.   Ford AC, Moayeddi P, Chey WD, et al. American College of Gastroenterology monograph on management of irritable bowel syndrome. *Am J Gastroenterol* 2018;113:1–18.

29.   Alammar N, Wang L, Saberi B, et al. The impact of peppermint oil on the irritable bowel syndrome: A meta-analysis of the pooled clinical data. *BMC Compliment Altern Med* 2019;19:21.

30.   Weerts ZZ, Masclee AAM, Witteman BJM, et al. Efficacy and safety of peppermint oil in a randomized, double-blink trial of patients with IBS. *Gastroenterol* 2020;158:123–36.

31.   Ford AC, Moayyedi P, Lacy BE, et al. American College of Gastroenterology monograph on the management of irritable bowel syndrome and chronic idiopathic constipation. *Am J Gastroenterol* 2014;109(Suppl 1):S2–26.

32.   Atluri DK, Chandar AK, Bharucha A, et al. Effect of linaclotide in irritable bowel syndrome with constipation (IBS-C)L a systematic review and meta-analysis. *Neurogastroenterol Motil* 2014;26:499–509.

33.   Shah ED, Kim HM, Schoenfeld P. Efficacy and tolerability of guanylate cyclase-c agonists for irritable bowel syndrome with constipation and chronic idiopathic constipation: A systematic review and meta-analysis. *Am J Gastroenterol* 2018;113:329–38.

34.   Xie C, Tang Y, Wang Y, et al. Efficacy and safety of antidepressants for the treatment of irritable bowel syndrome: A meta-analysis. *PLoS One* 2015;10:e0127815.

35.   Ford AC, Lacy BE, Harris L, et al. Effect of antidepressants and psychological therapies in irritable bowel syndrome: An updated systematic review and meta-analysis. *Am J Gastroenterol* 2019;114:21–39.

36.   Laird KT, Tanner-Smith EE, Russell AC, et al. Short-term and long-term efficacy of psychological therapies for irritable bowel syndrome: A systematic review and meta-analysis. *Clin Gastroenterol Hepatol* 2016;14:937–47 e934.

37.   Bianchi M, Festa V, Moretti A, Ciaco A, et al. Meta-analysis: long-term therapy with rifaximin in the management of uncomplicated diverticular disease. *Aliment Pharmacol Ther.* 2011;33:902-10.

38.   Strate LL, Modi R, Cohen E, Spiegel BMR. Diverticular disease as a chronic illness: evolving epidemiologic and clinical insights. *Am J. Gastroenterol.* 2012;107:1486-93.

39.   Alamo RZ, Quigley EMM. Irritable bowel syndrome and colonic diverticular disease: overlapping symptoms and overlapping therapeutic approaches. *Curr Opin Gastroenterol.* 2019;35:27-33.

40.   Ford AC, Harris LA, Lacy BE, et al. Systematic review with meta-analysis: The efficacy of prebiotics, probiotics, synbiotics and antibiotics in irritable bowel syndrome. *Aliment Pharmacol Ther* 2018;48:1044–60.

41.   Fodor AA, Pimentel M, Chey WD, et al. Rifaximin is associated with modest, transient decreases in multiple taxa in the gut microbiota of patients with diarrhoea-predominant irritable bowel syndrome. *Gut Microbes* 2019;10:22–33.

42.   Ford AC, Brandt LJ, Young C, et al. Efficacy of 5-HT3 antagonists and 5-HT4 agonists in irritable bowel syndrome: Systematic review and meta-analysis. *Am J Gastroenterol* 2009;104:1831–43.

43.   LeBrett WG, Chen FW, Yng L, Chang L. Increasing rates of opioid prescriptions for gastrointestinal diseases in the United States. *Am J Gastroenterol.* 2021;116:796-807

44.   Lembo AJ, Lacy BE, Zuckerman MJ, et al. Eluxadoline for irritable bowel syndrome with diarrhea. *N Engl J Med* 2016;374:242–53.

45.   Slattery SA, Niaz O, Aziz Q, et al. Systematic review with meta-analysis: The prevalence of bile acid malabsorption in the irritable bowel syndrome with diarrhoea. *Aliment Pharmacol* Ther 2015;42:3–11.

46.   Tack J, Carbone F, Holvoet L, Vanheel H, Vanuytsel T, Vandenberghe A. The use of pictograms improves symptom evaluation by patients with functional dyspepsia. *Aliment Pharmacol* Ther 2014;40:523–30.

47.   Moayyedi P, Lacy BE, Andrews CN, Enns RA, Howden CW, Vakil N. ACG and CAG clinical guideline: Management of Dyspepsia. *Am J Gastroenterol.* 2017;112:988-1013

48.   Cangemi DJ, Marilia M, Spiegel B, Lacy B. Virtual reality improves symptoms of functional dyspepsia: results of a randomized, double-blind, sham-controlled pilot study. *Am J Gastroenterol* 2023. In press.

49.   Kotikula I, Thinrungroj N, Pinyopornpanish K, et al. Randomised clinical trial: the effects of pregabalin vs placebo on functional dyspepsia. *Aliment Pharmacol Ther.* 2021;54:1026-1032

50.   Tack J, Giao Ly H, Carbone F, et al. Efficacy of mirtazapine in patients with functional dyspepsia and weight loss. *Clin Gastroenterol Hepatol* 2016;14:385-392

51.   Wald A, Bharucha AE, Limketkai B, Malcolm A, Remes-Troche JM, Whitehead WE, Massarat Z. ACG Clinical Guidelines: Management of Benign Anorectal Disorders. *Am J Gastroenterol.* 2021;116:1987-2008

52.   Spiegel B. *Acing the GI Board Exams, 2ⁿᵈ Edition.* Page 55. SLACK, Inc, Thorofare, NJ.

53.   Prott G, Shim L, Hansen R, et al. Relationships between pelvic floor symptoms and function in irritable bowel syndrome. Neurogastroenterol Motil 2010;22:764–9.

54.   Rao SSC. Rectal exam: Yes, it can and should be done in a busy practice! *Am J Gastroenterol.* 2018;113:635-638

55.   Tantiphlachiva K, Rao P, Attaluri A, et al. Digital rectal examination is a useful tool for identifying patients with dyssynergia. Clin Gastroenterol Hepatol 2010;8:955–60.

56.   Abbott R, Ayres I, Hui E, Hui Ka-Kit. Effect of perineal self-acupressure on constipation: a randomized controlled trial. *J Gen Intern Med.* 2015;30:434-439

57.   Rao S, Bharucha AE, Chiarioni G, et al. Functional anorectal disorders. Gastroenterology 2016;150:1430–42.

58.   Whitehead WE, Borrud L, Goode PS, et al. Fecal incontinence in US adults: Epidemiology and risk factors. *Gastroenterology* 2009;137:512–7.

59.   Nelson R, Furner S, Jesudason V. Fecal incontinence in Wisconsin nursing homes: Prevalence and associations. *Dis Colon Rectum* 1998;41:1226–9.

60.   Rao SSC, Benninga MA, Bharucha AE, Chiarioni G, Di Lorenzo C, Whitehead WE. AMNS-ESNM position paper and consensus guideline on biofeedback therapy for anorectal disorders. *Neurogastroenterol Motil.* 2015;27:594-609

61.   Leo CA, Thomas GP, Hodgkinson JD, et al. The Renew® anal insert for passive faecal incontinence: A retrospective audit of our use of a novel device. *Colorectal Dis* 2019;21:684–8.

62.   Richter HE, Matthews CA, Muir T, et al. A vaginal bowel-control system for the treatment of fecal incontinence. *Obstet Gynecol* 2015;125:540–7.

63.   Graf W, Mellgren A, Matzel KE, et al. Efficacy of dextranomer in stabilised hyaluronic acid for treatment of faecal incontinence: a randomised, sham-controlled trial. *The Lancet* 2011;377:997–1003.

64.   Camillero M, Kuo B, Nguyen L, et al. ACG clinical guideline: Gastroparesis. *Am J Gastroenterol* 2022;117:1197-1220

65.   Parkman HP, Wilson LA, Hasler WL, et al. Abdominal Pain in Patients with Gastroparesis: Associations with Gastroparesis Symptoms, Etiology of Gastroparesis, Gastric Emptying, Somatization, and Quality of Life. *Dig Dis Sci.* 2019;64:2242-2255

66.   Abell TL, Camilleri M, Donohoe K, et al. American Neurogastroenterology and motility Society and the Society of nuclear medicine consensus recommendations for gastric emptying scintigraphy: A joint report of the American Neurogastroenterology and motility Society and the Society of nuclear medicine. *Am J Gastroenterol* 2008;103:753–63.

67.   Camilleri M, Zinsmeister AR, Greydanus MP, Brown ML, Proano M. Towards a less costly but accurate test of gastric emptying and small bowel transit. *Dig Dis Sci.* 1991;36:609-15

68.   Pasricha PJ, Grover M, Yates KP, et al. Functional dyspepsia and gastroparesis in tertiary care are interchangeable syndromes with common clinical and pathologic features. *Gastroenterology* 2021;160: 2006–17.

69.   Viramontes BE, Kim DY, Camilleri M, et al. Validation of a stable isotope gastric emptying test for normal, accelerated or delayed gastric emptying. Neurogastroenterol Motil 2001;13:567–74.

70.   Olausson EA, Sto⊠rsrud S, Grundin H, et al. A small particle size diet reduces upper gastrointestinal symptoms in patients with diabetic gastroparesis: A randomized controlled trial. Am J Gastroenterol 2014; 109:375–85.

71.   Lee A, Kuo B. Metoclopramide in the treatment of diabetic gastroparesis. *Expert Rev Endocrinol Metab.* 2010;5(5):653-662. doi:10.1586/eem.10.41

72.   Rao AS, Camilleri M. Review article: metoclopramide and tardive dyskinesia. *Aliment Pharmacol Ther.* 2010;31:11-9

73.   Al-Saffar A, Lennerna⊠s H, Hellstro⊠m PM. Gastroparesis, metoclopramide, and tardive dyskinesia: Risk revisited. *Neurogastroenterol Motil* 2019;31:e13617.

74.   Reddymasu SC, Soykan I, McCallum RW. Domperidone: review of pharmacology and clinical applications in gastroenterology. *Am J Gastroenterol.* 2007;102:2036-45

75.   Thielemans L, Depoortere I, Perret J, et al. Desensitization of the human motilin receptor by motilides. *J Pharmacol Exp Ther* 2005;313:1397–405

76.   Gorelik E, Masarwa R, Perlman A, et al. Systematic Review, Meta- analysis, and network meta-analysis of the cardiovascular safety of macrolides. *Antimicrob Agents Chemother* 2018;62:e00438–18

77.   Carbone F, Van den Houte K, Clevers E, et al. Prucalopride in gastroparesis: A randomized placebo-controlled crossover study. *Am J Gastroenterol* 2019;114:1265–74

78.   Tack J, Rotondo A, Meulemans A, et al. Randomized clinical trial: A controlled pilot trial of the 5-HT4 receptor agonist revexepride in patients with symptoms suggestive of gastroparesis. *Neurogastroenterol Motil* 2016;28:487–97

79.   Chang L, Chey WD, Imdad A, et al. American Gastroenterological Association-American College of Gastroenterology Clinical Practice Guideline: Pharmacological Management of Chronic Idiopathic Constipation. *Am J Gastroenterol* 2023 (in press)

80.   McRorie J, Fahey G, Gibb RD, et al. Laxative effects of wheat bran and psyllium: Resolving enduring misconceptions about fiber in treatment guidelines for chronic idiopathic constipation. *J Am Assoc Nurse Pract* 2020;32(1):15–23.

81.   Dipalma JA, Cleveland MV, McGowan J, et al. A randomized, multicenter, placebo-controlled trial of polyethylene glycol laxative for chronic treatment of chronic constipation. Am J Gastroenterol 2007; 102(7):1436–41.

82.   Cinca R, Chera D, Gruss HJ, et al. Randomised clinical trial: macrogol/ PEG 3350 electrolytes versus prucalopride in the treatment of chronic constipation: A comparison in a controlled environment. Aliment Pharmacol Ther 2013;37(9):876–86.

83.   Di Palma JA, Cleveland MV, McGowan J, et al. A randomized, multicenter comparison of polyethylene glycol laxative and tegaserod in treatment of patients with chronic constipation. Am J Gastroenterol 2007; 102(9):1964–71.

84.   Katz PO, Dunbar KB, Schnoll-Sussman FH, et al. ACG Clinical Guideline for the Diagnosis and Management of Gastroesophageal Reflux Disease. *Am J Gastroenterol* 2021;117:27-56

85.   Cremonini F, Wise J, Moayyedi P, et al. Diagnostic and therapeutic use of proton pump inhibitors in non-cardiac chest pain: A metaanalysis. Am J Gastroenterol 2005;100(6):1226–32.

86.   Ness-Jensen E, Lindam A, Lagergren J, et al. Tobacco smoking cessation and improved gastroesophageal reflux: A prospective population-based cohort study: The HUNT study. *Am J Gastroenterol* 2014;109(2):171–7.

87. El-Serag H, Becher A, Jones R. Systematic review: Persistent reflux symptoms on proton pump inhibitor therapy in primary care and community studies. Aliment Pharmacol Ther 2010;32(6):720–37.

88. Fass R, Sontag SJ, Traxler B, et al. Treatment of patients with persistent heartburn symptoms: A double-blind, randomized trial. *Clin Gastroenterol Hepatol* 2006;4(1):50–6

89. Gralnek IM, Dulai GS, Fennerty MB, Spiegel BMR. Esomeprazole versus other proton pump inhibitors in erosive esophagitis: A meta-analysis of randomized clinical trials. *Clin Gastroenterol Hepatol* 2006;4(12):1452–8.

90. Spechler SJ, Hunter JG, Jones KM, et al. Randomized trial of medical versus surgical treatment for refractory heartburn. *N Engl J Med* 2019; 381(16):1513–23.

91. Rickenbacher N, Kötter T, Kochen MM, et al. Fundoplication versus medical management of gastroesophageal reflux disease: Systematic review and meta-analysis. Surg Endosc 2014;28(1):143–55.

92. Garg SK, Gurusamy KS. Laparoscopic fundoplication surgery versus medical management for gastro-oesophageal reflux disease (GORD) in adults. Cochrane Database Syst Rev 2015(11):CD003243.

93. Ganz RA, Peters JH, Horgan S, et al. Esophageal sphincter device for gastroesophageal reflux disease. *N Engl J Med* 2013;368(8):719–27.

94. Alicuben ET, Bell RCW, Jobe BA, et al. Worldwide experience with erosion of the magnetic sphincter augmentation device. *J Gastrointest Surg* 2018;22(8):1442–7.

95. Bell R, Lipham J, Louie B, et al. Magnetic sphincter augmentation superior to proton pump inhibitors for regurgitation in a 1-year randomized trial. *Clin Gastroenterol Hepatol* 2020;18(8):1736–43.e2.

96. Lipka S, Kumar A, Richter JE. No evidence for efficacy of radiofrequency ablation for treatment of gastroesophageal reflux disease: A systematic review and meta-analysis. *Clin Gastroenterol Hepatol* 2015;13(6):1058–67.e1.

97. Hunter JG, Kahrilas PJ, Bell RCW, et al. Efficacy of transoral fundoplication vs omeprazole for treatment of regurgitation in a randomized controlled trial. *Gastroenterology* 2015;148(2):324–33.e5.

98. McCarty TR, Itidiare M, Njei B, et al. Efficacy of transoral incisionless fundoplication for refractory gastroesophageal reflux disease: A systematic review and meta-analysis. *Endoscopy* 2018;50(7):708–25.

99. Testoni S, Hassan C, Mazzoleni G, et al. Long-term outcomes of transoral incisionless fundoplication for gastro-esophageal reflux disease: Systematic- review and meta-analysis. Endosc Int Open 2021;9(2):E239–e246.

100. Shaheen NJ, Crosby MA, Bozymski EM, Sandler RS. Is there publication bias in the reporting of cancer risk in Barrett's esophagus? *Gastroenterol* 2000;119:333-8

101. Shaheen N, Falk GW, Prasad I, et al. Diagnosis and management of Barrett's esophagus: An upated ACG guideline. *Am J Gastroenterol* 2022;117:559-587

102. Qumseya BJ, Bukannan A, Gendy S, et al. Systematic review and metaanalysis of prevalence and risk factors for Barrett's esophagus. Gastrointest Endosc 2019;90:707–17

103. Shaheen NJ, Dulai G, Ascher B, Mitchell K, Schmitz SM. Effect of a new diagnosis of Barrett's esophagus on insurance status. *Am J Gastroenterol* 2005;100:577-80

104. 104   Wani S, Williams JW, Falk GW, et al. An analysis of the GIQuIC nationwide quality registry reveals unnecessary surveillance endoscopies in patients with normal and irregular Z-lines. *Am J Gastroenterol* 2020;115:1869-1878

105. Sharma P, Dent J, Armstrong A, et al. The development and validation of an endoscopic grading system for Barrett's esophagus: the Prague C&M criteria. *Am J Gastroenterol* 2006;131:1392-9

106. Dellon E, Gonsalves N, Hirano I, et al. ACG clinical guideline: evidence based approach to the diagnosis and management of esophageal eosinophilia and eosinophilic esophagitis (EoE). *Am J Gastroenterol* 2013;108:679-692

107. Hirano I, Chan ES, Rank MA, et al. AGA Institute and the Joint Task Force on Allergy-Immunology Practice Parameters Clinical Guidelines for the Management of Eosinophilic Esophagitis. *Gastroenterol* 2020;158:1776-1786

108. Hirano I, Moy N, Heckman MG, Thomas CS, Gonsalves N, Achem SR. Endoscopic assessment of the oesophageal features of eosinophilic oesophagitis: validation of a novel classification and grading system. Gut. 2013;62(4):489-495. doi:10.1136/gutjnl-2011-301817

109. Muller S, Puhl S, Vieth M *et al*. Analysis of symptoms and endoscopic findings in 117 patients with histological diagnoses of eosinophilic esophagitis. Endoscopy 2007;39:339–344.

110. Lucendo AJ, Arias A, Molina-Infante J. Efficacy of proton pump inhibitor drugs for inducing clinical and histological remission in patients with symptomatic esophageal eosinophilia: a systematic review and meta-analysis. *Clin Gastroenterol Hepatol.* 2016;14:13-22.e1

111. Alexander JA, Jung KW, Arora AS *et al*. Swallowed fluticasone improves histologic but not symptomatic responses of adults with eosinophilic esophagitis. Clin Gastroenterol Hepatol 2012;10:742–749. e1.

112. Arora AS, Perrault J, Smyrk TC. Topical corticosteroid treatment of dysphagia due to eosinophilic esophagitis in adults. Mayo Clin Proc 2003;78:830–835.

113. Lucendo AJ, De Rezende LC, Jimenez-Contreras S *et al*. Montelukast was inefficient in maintaining steroid-induced remission in adult eosinophilic esophagitis. Dig Dis Sci 2011;56:3551–3558.

114. Dellon ES, Rothenberg ME, Collins MH, et al. Dupilumab in adults and adolescents with eosinophilic esophagitis. *N Engl J Med.* 2022;387:2317-2330

115. Vaezi MF, Pandolfino JE, Yadlapati RH, et al. ACG clinical guidelines: diagnosis and management of achalasia. *Am J Gastroenterol* 2020;115:1393-1411

116. Pandolfino JE, Kwiatek MA, Nealis T, et al. Achalasia: A new clinically relevant classification by high-resolution manometry. *Gastroenterology* 2008;135(5):1526–33.

117. Hirano I, Pandolfino JE, Boeckxstaens GE. Functional lumen imaging probe for the management of esophageal disorders: Expert review from the Clinical Practice Updates Committee of the AGA Institute. Clin Gastroenterol Hepatol 2017;15(3):325–34

118. Eckardt VF, Kanzler G, Westermeier T. Complications and their impact after pneumatic dilation for achalasia: Prospective long-term follow-up study. Gastrointest Endosc 1997;45(5):349–53.

119. Evensen H, Kristensen V, Larssen L, et al. Outcome of peroral endoscopic myotomy (POEM) in treatment-naive patients. A systematic review. Scand J Gastroenterol 2019;54(1):1–7.

120. Shergill J, Makaroff KE, Lauzon M, Spiegel BMR, Almario CV. Fecal immunochemical test (FIT) versus colonoscopy: Does knowing that a positive FIT requires follow-up colonoscopy affect initial decision making in the US? *Prev Med Rep.* 2022;13:27:101825

121. Robertson D, Lee Jeffrey, Boland R, et al. Recommendations on fecal immunochemical testing to screen for colorectal neoplasia: A consensus statement by the US Multi-Society Task Force on Colorectal Cancer. *Am J Gastroenterol* 2017;112:37-53

122. Lee JK, Liles EG, Bent S *et al*. Accuracy of fecal immunochemical tests for colorectal cancer: systematic review and meta-analysis. Ann Intern Med 2014;160:171.

123. Quintero E, Castells A, Bujanda L *et al*. Colonoscopy versus fecal immunochemical testing in colorectal-cancer screening. *N Engl J Med* 2012;366:697–706.

124. Imperiale TF, Ransohoff DF, Itzkowitz SH, et al. Multitarget stool DNA testing for colorectal-cancer screening. *N Engl J Med* 2014;370:1287-97

125. Cotter TG, Burger KN, Devens ME, et al. Long-term follow-up of patients having false-positive multitarget stool DNA tests after negative screening colonoscopy: The LONG-HAUL cohort study. Cancer Epidemiol Biomarkers Prev 2017;26:614–21.

126. Berger BM, Kisiel JB, Imperiale TF, et al. Low incidence of aerodigestive cancers in patients with negative results from colonoscopies, regardless of findings from multitarget stool DNA tests. Clin Gastroenterol Hepatol 2020;18:864–71.

127. Shaukat A, Kahi CJ, Burke CA, Rabeneck L, Sauer BG, Rex DK. ACG Clinical Guidelines: Colorectal Cancer Screening 2021. Am J Gastroenterol. 2021 Mar 1;116(3):458-479.

128. Lee SJ, Boscardin WJ, Stijacic-Cenzer I, et al. Time lag to benefit after screening for breast and colorectal cancer: meta-analysis of survival data from the United States, Sweden, United Kingdom, and Denmark. BMJ 2013;346:e8441.

129. U.S. Preventive Services Task Force. Screening for colorectal cancer: Recommendations and rationale. Ann Intern Med 2002;137: 129–31.

130. Imperiale TF, Ransohoff DF. Risk for colorectal cancer in persons with a family history of adenomatous polyps: A systematic review. Ann Intern Med 2012;156:703–9.

131. Ng SC, Lau JY, Chan FK, et al. Risk of advanced adenomas in siblings of individuals with advanced adenomas: A cross-sectional study. Gastroenterology 2016;150:608–16; quiz e16–7.

132. Click B, Pinsky PF, Hickey T, et al. Association of colonoscopy adenoma findings with long-term colorectal cancer Laiyemo Lincidence. JAMA 2018;319:2021–2031.

133. Dube C, Yakubu M, McCurdy BR, et al. Risk of advanced adenoma, colorectal cancer, and colorectal cancer mortality in people with low-risk adenomas at baseline colonoscopy: a systematic review and metaanalysis. Am J Gastroenterol 2017;112:1790–1801.

134. Knudsen AB, Hur C, Gazelle GS, et al. Rescreening of persons with a negative colonoscopy result: results from a microsimulation model. Ann Intern Med 2012;157:611–620.

135. Gupta S, Lieberman D, Anderson JC, et al. Recommendations for Follow-Up After Colonoscopy and Polypectomy: A Consensus Update by the US Multi-Society Task Force on Colorectal Cancer. *Am J Gastroenterol.* 2020 Mar;115(3):415-434.

136. Belderbos TD, Leenders M, Moons LM, et al. Local recurrence after endoscopic mucosal resection of nonpedunculated colorectal lesions: systematic review and meta-analysis. Endoscopy 2014;46:388–402.

137. Pellise M, Burgess NG, Tutticci N, et al. Endoscopic mucosal resection for large serrated lesions in comparison with adenomas: a prospective multicentre study of 2000 lesions. Gut 2017;66:644–653.

138. Rex KD, Vemulapalli KC, Rex DK. Recurrence rates after EMR of large sessile serrated polyps. Gastrointest Endosc 2015;82:538–541.

139. Pohl H, Srivastava A, Bensen SP, et al. Incomplete polyp resection during colonoscopy-results of the complete adenoma resection (CARE) study. Gastroenterology 2013;144:74–80.e1.

140. Kaltenbach TA, Anderson JC, Burke CA, et al. Endoscopic removal of colorectal lesions—recommendations by the US Multi-Society Task Force on Colorectal Cancer. Am J Gastroenterol 2020;115(3):435-464.

141. Benson AB, Venook AP, Al-Hawary MM, et al. Colon Cancer, Version 2. 2021, NCCN Clinical Practice Guidelines in Oncology. *J Natl Compr Canc Netw.* 2021 Mar 2;19(3):329-359.

142. Johnson DA, Barkun A, Cohen LB, et al. Optimizing adequacy of bowel cleansing for colonoscopy: Recommendations from the US Multi-Society Task Force on Colorectal Cancer. *Am J Gastroenterol* 2014;109:1528-1545

143. Abuksis G, Mor M, Segal N et al. A patient education program is cost-effective for preventing failure of endoscopic procedures in a gastroenterology department. Am J Gastroenterol 2001; 96: 1786 – 90.

144. Spiegel BMR, Talley J, Shekelle P, et al. Development and validation of a novel patient educational booklet to enhance colonoscopy preparation. *Am J Gastroenterol* 2011;106:875-83

145. Siddiqui AA, Yang K, Spechler SJ et al. Duration of the interval between the completion of bowel preparation and the start of colonoscopy predicts bowel-preparation quality. Gastrointest Endosc 2009; 69: 700 – 6.

146. Jover R, Zapater P, Polania E et al. Modifiable endoscopic factors that influence the adenoma detection rate in colorectal cancer screening colonoscopies. Gastrointest Endosc 2013; 77: 381 – 9.

147. Longcroft -Wheaton G, Bhandari P. Same-day bowel cleansing regimen is superior to a split-dose regimen over two days for afternoon colonoscopy: results from a large prospective series. J Clin Gastroenterol 2012; 46: 57 – 61.

148. Zauber AG, Winawer SJ, O'Brien MJ, et al. Colonoscopic polypectomy and long-term prevention of colorectal-cancer deaths. N Engl J Med 2012;366:687–696.

149. Kaltenbach T, Anderson JC, Burke CA, et al. Endoscopic removal of colorectal lesions: recommendations by the US Multi-Society Task Force on Colorectal Cancer. *Am J Gastroenterol* 2020;115:435-464

150. Barclay RL, Vicari JJ, Greenlaw RL. Effect of a time-dependent colonoscopic withdrawal protocol on adenoma detection during screening colonoscopy. Clin Gastroenterol Hepatol 2008;6:1091–1098.

151. Reg DK, Schoenfeld PS, Cohen J, et al. Quality indicators for colonoscopy. *Am J Gastroenterol* 2015;110:72-90

152. Soetikno RM, Kaltenbach T, Rouse RV, et al. Prevalence of nonpolypoid (flat and depressed) colorectal neoplasms in asymptomatic and symptomatic adults. JAMA 2008;299:1027–1035.

153. Bogie RMM, Veldman MHJ, Snijders LARS, et al. Endoscopic subtypes of colorectal laterally spreading tumors (LSTs) and the risk of submucosal invasion: a meta-analysis. Endoscopy 2018;50:263–282.

154. Hewett DG, Kaltenbach T, Sano Y, et al. Validation of a simple classification system for endoscopic diagnosis of small colorectal polyps using narrow-band imaging. Gastroenterology 2012;143:599–607.e1.

155. Kudo S, Tamura S, Nakajima T, et al. Diagnosis of colorectal tumorous lesions by magnifying endoscopy. Gastrointest Endosc 1996;44:8–14.

156. Swan MP, Bourke MJ, Moss A, Williams SJ, Hopper A, Metz A. The target sign: an endoscopic marker for the resection of the muscularis propria and potential perforation during colonic endoscopic mucosal resection. Gastrointest Endosc. 2011 Jan;73(1):79-85.

157. Pohl H, Grimm IS, Moyer MT, et al. Clip closure prevents bleeding after endoscopic resection of large colon polyps in a randomized trial. Gastroenterology 2019 Oct;157:977–984.

158. Bahin FF, Naidoo M, Williams SJ, et al. Prophylactic endoscopic coagulation to prevent bleeding after wide-field endoscopic mucosal resection of large sessile colon polyps. Clin Gastroenterol Hepatol 2015; 13:724–730 e1–e2.

159. Syngal S, Brand RE, Church JM, et al. ACG Clinical Guideline: Genetic Testing and Management of Hereditary Gastrointestinal Cancer Syndromes. *Am J Gastroenterol* 2015;110:223-262

160. Giardiello FM, Allen JI, Axilbund JE, et al. Guidelines on Genetic Evaluation and Management of Lynch Syndrome: A Consensus Statement by the US Multi-Society Task Force on Colrectal Cancer. *Am J Gastroenterol* 2014;109:1159-1179

161. Kahi CJ, Boland CR, Dominitz JA, et al. Colonoscopy surveillance after colorectal cancer resection: Recommendations of the US Multi-Society Task Force on Colorectal Cancer. *Am J Gastroenterol.* 2016;111:337-46

162. Park SH, Lee JH, Lee SS et al. CT colonography for detection and characterization of synchronous proximal colonic lesions in patients with stenosing colorectal cancer. Gut 2012; 61: 1716 – 22.

163. Halligan S, Wooldrage K, Dadswell E et al. Computed tomographic colonography versus barium enema for diagnosis of colorectal cancer or large polyps in symptomatic patients (SIGGAR): a multicentre randomized trial. Lancet 2013; 381: 1185 – 93.

164. Levin B, Lieberman DA, McFarland B et al. Screening and surveillance for the early detection of colorectal cancer and adenomatous polyps, 2008: a joint guideline from the American Cancer Society, the US Multi-Society Task Force on Colorectal Cancer, and the American College of Radiology. Gastroenterology 2008; 134: 1570 – 95.

165. Renehan AG, Egger M, Saunders MP et al. Impact on survival of intensive follow up after curative resection for colorectal cancer: systematic review and meta-analysis of randomised trials. BMJ 2002; 324: 813.

166. Singh A, Kuo YF, Goodwin JS. Many patients who undergo surgery for colorectal cancer receive surveillance colonoscopies earlier than recommended by guidelines. Clin Gastroenterol Hepatol 2013; 11: 65 – 72 e1

167. Kapiteijn E, Marijnen CA, Nagtegaal ID et al. Preoperative radiotherapy combined with total mesorectal excision for resectable rectal cancer. N Engl J Med 2001; 345: 638 – 46.

168. Pfister DG, Benson AB 3rd, Somerfield MR. Clinical practice. Surveillance strategies after curative treatment of colorectal cancer. N Engl J Med 2004; 350: 2375 – 82.

169. Jacobson BC, Bhatt A, Greer KB et al. ACG Clinical Guideline: Diagnosis and Management of Gastrointestinal Subepithelial Lesions. *Am J Gastroenterol* 2023;18:46-58

170. Faigel DO, Abullhawa S. Gastrointestinal stromal tumors: The role of the gastroenterologist in diagnosis and risk stratification. *J Clin Gastroenterol* 2012;46:629-36

171. Rindi G, Luinetti O, Cornaggia M, et al. Three subtypes of gastric argyrophil carcinoid and the gastric neuroendocrine carcinoma: A clinicopathologic study. Gastroenterology 1993;104:994–1006

www.ingramcontent.com/pod-product-compliance
Lightning Source LLC
Chambersburg PA
CBHW041156150726
48006CB00016B/2003